AF614693

Family Therapy - Recent Advances in Clinical and Crisis Settings

Edited by Oluwatoyin Olatundun Ilesanmi

Published in London, United Kingdom

Family Therapy - Recent Advances in Clinical and Crisis Settings
http://dx.doi.org/10.5772/intechopen.102131
Edited by Oluwatoyin Olatundun Ilesanmi

Contributors
Lucy C Parker-Barnes, Noel McKillip, Carolyn Powell, Maliha Ibrahim, Manjushree Palit, Rhea Matthews, Barry Viljoen, Oluwatoyin Olatundun Ilesanmi, Faith Ibitoyosi Ilesanmi, Raouf Hajji

First published in London, United Kingdom, 2023 by IntechOpen
IntechOpen is the global imprint of INTECHOPEN LIMITED, registered in England and Wales, registration number: 11086078, 5 Princes Gate Court, London, SW7 2QJ, United Kingdom

British Library Cataloguing-in-Publication Data
A catalogue record for this book is available from the British Library

Additional hard and PDF copies can be obtained from orders@intechopen.com

Family Therapy - Recent Advances in Clinical and Crisis Settings
Edited by Oluwatoyin Olatundun Ilesanmi
p. cm.
Print ISBN 978-1-83769-989-6
Online ISBN 978-1-83768-214-0
eBook (PDF) ISBN 978-1-83768-215-7

For EU product safety concerns:
IN TECH d.o.o., Prolaz Marije Krucifikse Kozulić 3, 51000 Rijeka, Croatia,
info@intechopen.com or visit our website at intechopen.com.

Meet the editor

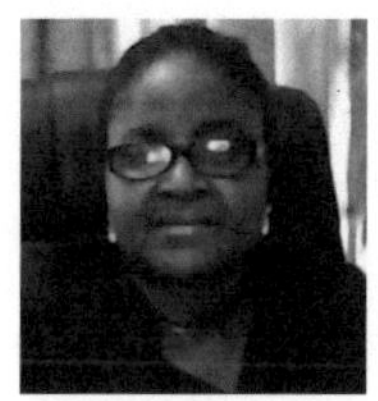

Dr. Oluwatoyin Olatundun Ilesanmi obtained an MEd in Guidance Counselling and a Ph.D. in Clinical Psychology from the University of Ibadan, Nigeria in 2005 and 1999, respectively. She is an associate professor at the Centre for Gender, Humanitarian and Development Studies, Redeemer's University, Ede, Osun State, Nigeria. Dr. Ilesanmi is a clinical humanitarian psychologist, a genetic counsellor, and a gender and development expert with core competencies in research, evidence-based programming, policy analysis and guidelines development, psychosocial management of sickle cell disorders, gender equality and socially inclusive research, consultancies and initiatives related to sexual harassment and gender-based violence (SH/GBV,) multi-sectoral GESI inclusive programming and strategic planning, and mainstreaming gender equality and empowerment of women and girls (GEEWG) into the humanitarian system.

Contents

Preface

We live in a time of unprecedented humanitarian emergencies, many of which have been created and exacerbated by natural disasters, insurgencies, and armed conflict. Individual and family resilience is the ability of the family to rebound from life crises and persistent humanitarian challenges. Family systems therapy has become an essential framework to understand human functioning and dysfunction in humanitarian catastrophes. It is a well-recognized psychotherapeutic approach aimed at the family system. Its practice has evolved across geographical locations since the early 1950s.

Clinically, family therapy developed within the context of several therapeutic movements, including child guidance clinics, marriage counselling, and sex therapy. Whilst it is theoretically rooted in the interdisciplinary field of systems theory, or cybernetics, systemic family therapy has prided itself on its usefulness in humanitarian settings or following the onset of the humanitarian crisis.

Family Therapy – Recent Advances in Clinical and Crisis Settings explores the structural, social constructionism, and solution-focused brief approaches to systemic family therapy. It regards the family context in humanitarian settings as being of paramount significance for an individual's psychological development and emotional well-being. The book examines how the family interacts as a cohesive unit during humanitarian catastrophes and looks at patterns among individuals that influence or impede the potential for change within the family system.

The scope of the book is within the context of global complex humanitarian catastrophes and encompasses cross-cutting contemporary issues and mental health challenges pertaining to violence, loss of loved ones and properties, rape and other forms of sexual assault, displacement, poverty, discrimination, overcrowding, disconnection from previous sources of social support and food, resource insecurity, migration, sexuality and reproduction concerns, sexual orientation and gender identity, conflict, socioeconomic concerns, disabilities, widespread anxiety, fear, and hardship for the affected persons and their families.

Family Therapy – Recent Advances in Clinical and Crisis Settings also explores the processes and practices of family systems therapy as conducted in humanitarian situations across the globe. It provides readers with a comprehensive overview of the current state-of-the-art innovative advances in family counselling and psychotherapies for families and couples in humanitarian crises, conflicts, and disasters.

Included in the book are scholarly chapters by researchers, students, professionals, and trainees from diverse locales that document remarkable examples of courage and resilience on the part of therapists as well as clients within the context of humanitarian catastrophes.

The book includes the following chapters:

Chapter 1: "Introductory Chapter: Family Therapy – Recent Advances in Clinical and Crisis Settings"

Chapter 2: "Innovative Family Therapy for Households in Global Complex Humanitarian Crises"

Chapter 3: "Perspective Chapter: Theoretical Paradigm for Mental Health and Family Therapy within the South African Context – An Overview"

Chapter 4: "Perspective Chapter: Helping BIPOC LGBTQIA+ Families through Inclusive Therapy and Advocacy"

Chapter 5: "Intergenerational Attachment Styles, Emotional Regulation and Relational Outcomes in Couples Therapy"

The book explores recent advances in strengths-based therapies and contemporary models such as solution-focused, narrative, and conversational therapies for family relationships. It is highly relevant and useful for professionals, clients and patients, policymakers, decision-makers in healthcare delivery, and representatives of public and private health insurance schemes.

Oluwatoyin Olatundun Ilesanmi
Centre for Gender,
Humanitarian and Development Studies,
Redeemer's University,
Ede, Osun State, Nigeria

Chapter 1

Introductory Chapter: Family Therapy – Recent Advances in Clinical and Crisis Settings

Oluwatoyin Olatundun Ilesanmi

1. Introduction

Promoting recent advances in family therapy for the psychosocial strengthening of bonding, cohesion, healing, and behavior modification in response to adversity in clinical settings is a burning global public and mental health concern. Families are an important part of the social fabric and support system as well as an integral part of the psychological treatment and therapeutic processes involved in the management of individuals with mental illness potentially induced by traumatic events such as the loss of loved ones, disasters, accidents, addiction, and other causes. Family reactions and dysfunctional responses to disastrous events and catastrophes may induce the risk of anxiety, depression, distress, trauma, post-traumatic stress symptoms, and emotional and behavioral problems in individuals and may also lower the capacity for resilience and adjustment [1].

Families are sociological constructs for the level of relationships classified as parent to parent, parent to child, and sibling to sibling in immediate families and through even more combinations in extended families. Moos and Moos [2] characterized families by their structure, roles, and boundaries: emotional bonds and responsiveness, cohesiveness, flexibility, adaptability, and coping, communication, and decision-making and problem-solving. Typically, families are set up to support, nurture, and protect members all through life, especially within the context of disasters.

Individual psychological problems such as depression and anxiety, psychoses, child and adolescent-related problems, and alcohol use disorders also affect their families too. The emotional consequences and psychosocial burden of an individual's mental illness on family members and caregivers may include courtesy stigma or stigma by association, which is the stigma that family members experience because of their association with a loved one who suffers from drug addiction or other forms of mental illness [3]. Beside experiencing stigma associated with mental illness, other forms of stigma include those that are associated with physical deformation and those that are attached to race, ethnicity, religion, and ideology.

Family therapy interventions are needed to reduce the emotional consequences, the psychosocial and economic burden of psychological illness, depression, and associated psychosis related to humanitarian catastrophes, BIPOC LGBTQIA+, marital stress, domestic violence, spousal abandonment and neglect, divorce and intimate partner violence (IPV), among other.

Consequently, this chapter explores the importance of this book titled "Family Therapy – Recent Advances in Clinical and Crisis Settings." It identifies categories of crisis setting in which family therapies could be applied. It highlighted MedFT and BSFT as *viable* options for the psychosocial management of families in crisis.

2. Importance of this book

The book titled "Family Therapy – Recent Advances in Clinical and Crisis Settings" is unique in its presentation of recent innovative advances in the terrain of global humanitarian catastrophes, clinical and crisis settings, BIPOC LGBTQIA+ settings, and couple counseling settings. Each of the articles presented in this book highlighted varying forms of family therapy including supportive family therapy (SFP), cognitive-behavioral therapy (CBT), psychodynamic therapies, and systemic family therapy.

Supportive family therapy often provides opportunities for therapists to offer practical advice in a safe and open environment for family members to openly express their feelings and talk about the issues affecting them. CBT provides opportunities for therapists to assign homework tasks or draw up specific behavioral programs for each individual family member to complete in order to change their negative thought patterns and behavior. Psychodynamic ideas are used in family therapy in order to address the individual's unconscious or subconscious mind so as to reduce the problem(s) by uncovering the underlying problems. SFP focuses attention on the entire family's feelings, ideas, and attitudes to identify the problems within a family dynamic and attempt to shift the problem(s), attitudes, and relationships to a position that is more beneficial, less damaging, or simply more realistic.

3. Categories of crisis settings of medical family therapy projected in this book

Family therapy often provides valuable opportunities for promoting growth and change that may result in the resolution of personal dysfunctional behaviors and family problems. Thus, this thought-provoking book shows that family therapy can be implemented in a range of settings including:

- **Home-based Setting:** The home-based family therapy (HBFT) is offered by clinicians and other mental health professionals to clients, family members, and other significant persons at their places of residence [4].

- **Global Humanitarian Catastrophes Settings:** This setting is appropriate for the delivery of couple and family therapy (CFT) intervention, especially through relational telehealth platforms.

- **Clinical Settings:** This implies the utilization of family therapy in the psychiatric scene. As Ackerman [5] puts it, an individual mental illness is an expression of symptoms of chronic pathology within the family as a whole. Effective intervention would, thus, require the inclusion of the entire family members in the treatment process.

- **Family Crisis Settings:** Psychopathology of the family system is a sign of dysfunctionality within the family system. Walsh [6] opines that "how families view their problems and their options can make all the difference between coping, healing, and growth or dysfunction, and despair. Beliefs that we are unworthy can fuel self-loathing, destructive behavior, or social isolation [6]." Thus, MedFT and BSFT are very apt treatment options for families in crisis.

- **BIPOC LGBTQIA+ Settings:** Malpas, Pellicane [7] opines that transgender and gender expansive (TGE) individuals sometimes are sometimes faced with disproportionate and challenging mental health and developmental outcomes. They also posit that family acceptance of TGE individuals' gender identity, and expression is crucial to preventing poor psychosocial outcomes and advocated for family-based therapies that will provide psychoeducation; enhance the protective power of family acceptance and provide opportunities for family members to express their reactions to TGE, gain allyship and advocacy, and connect with TGE community resources.

- **Couple Counseling Settings:** Systemic family therapy is useful for helping families and couples in intimate relationships to gain a deeper understanding of their interactions with each other: manage and resolve marital conflicts, communication problems, sex issues, anger, illness and stress, and nurture change and development [8].

4. Medical family therapy (MedFT) and brief strategic family therapy (BSFT) for families in clinical settings

Medical family therapy (MedFT) and brief strategic family therapy (BSFT) are forms of short-term counseling psychotherapies designed for assisting family members to improve communication with partners, children, or other family members and to resolve conflicts in troubled and dysfunctional relationships. According to Doherty and McDaniel [9], MedFT and BSFT are premised on the belief that all health and relationship problems are biological, psychological, and social in nature. MedFT and BSFT are active, directive, and task-oriented therapies, which include a range of psychoeducation, counseling, and coping skills.

Medical family therapy, (MedFT) and BSFT, are systemic biopsychosocial metaframeworks by which clinicians provide therapeutic services to patients and their families who are experiencing physical health problems [4]. With MedFTs and BSFT, the families are conceptualized holistically, while clinicians help family members to develop a sense of agency and communion to improve their lived experience.

MedFT and BSFT are usually provided by accredited psychologists, clinical social workers, or licensed therapists. The therapy sessions are often designed to address issues such as marital or financial problems, the conflict between parents and children, or the impact of substance abuse or a mental illness on the entire family. It may also be useful in teaching skills to deepen family connections and get through stressful times.

Zubatsky, Harris [10] and Szapocznik, and Schwartz [11] claimed that the main objective of MedFT and BSFT is the promotion of healing and well-being of clients and their family members. It aims at strengthening family cohesion and emotional bonds among family members, and their adaptability or capacity to adjust the family power structure, the structural interaction patterns, roles, and norms, which make up the family environment [1]. Through the exploration of agency and communion, MedFT and BSFT may be used to create a better home environment, solve family issues, and understand the unique issues that a family might face in diverse circumstances, especially during humanitarian catastrophes [12]. MedFTs and BSFT assist family members to develop a sense of agency in order to identify and develop strategies for managing what is within and outside of their control in regard to the illness experience [9].

Communion refers to one's connection and quality of social relationships with others [13]. MedFTs and BSFT assist clients and their families to develop strong communion through psychotherapeutic guidance for the creation and utilization of effective coping tools with the illness, thereby resulting in increasing connectedness, a sense of being cared for, loved for, and supported by each other [9].

MedFT and BSFT sessions are short-term models that typically consist of 12 to 17 weekly sessions, depending on the severity of the presenting problem. A typical session lasts 60 to 90 minutes. Both MedFTs and BSFTs utilize techniques such as joining, tracking and diagnosing, and restructuring to understand and change problematic family dynamics and behaviors.

Other forms of family therapy are Bowenian family therapy, communication family therapy, family systems therapy, functional family therapy, narrative family therapy, psychoeducation, structural family therapy, supportive family therapy, systemic therapy and transgenerational therapy.

5. Conclusion

In crisis settings, family therapy is advantageous in maintaining and building strong family cohesion, as well as for creating healthy and functional family relationships. These are conditions necessary for the creation of good psychological health and the elimination of psychopathological conditions within the family system. Medical family therapy and brief strategic family therapy are solution-focused and short-term therapies designed to help families going through any form of stressful events that may pull strain on their relationships. Examples of such stressful events are financial hardship, divorce, the death of a loved one, violent conflicts, and vulnerability to natural disasters.

Author details

Oluwatoyin Olatundun Ilesanmi
Centre for Gender and Humanitarian and Development Studies, Redeemer's University, Ede, Osun State, Nigeria

*Address all correspondence to: ilesanmit@run.edu.ng

References

[1] Walsh F. Family Therapy: Systemic Approaches to Practice, in Theory and Practice in Clinical Social Work, 2nd ed. Thousand Oaks, CA, US: Sage Publications, Inc; 2011. pp. 153-178

[2] Moos RH, Moos BS. A typology of family social environments. Journal of Family process. 1976;**15**(4):357-371

[3] Östman M, Kjellin L. Stigma by association: Psychological factors in relatives of people with mental illness. Journal of The British Journal of Psychiatry. 2002;**181**(6):494-498

[4] Finney N, Tadros E. Medical family therapy in home-based settings: A case application. The Family Journal. 2020;**28**(1):56-62

[5] Ackerman NW. Adolescent problems: A symptom of family disorder. Journal of Family Process. 1962;**1**(2):202-213. DOI: 10.1111/j.1545-5300.1962.00202.x

[6] Walsh F. Strengthening Family Resilience, 3rd ed. New York, NY, US: Guilford Press; 2016. p. xvi, 400-xvi, 400

[7] Malpas J, Pellicane MJ, Glaeser E. Family-based interventions with transgender and gender expansive youth: Systematic review and best practice recommendations. Journal of Transgender Health. 2022;**7**(1):7-29

[8] Lebow JL, Gurman AS. Research assessing couple and family therapy. Journal of Annual review of psychology. 1995;**46**(1):27-57

[9] Doherty WJ, McDaniel SH, Hepworth J. Contributions of medical family therapy to the changing health care system. Journal of Family Process. 2014;**53**(3):529-543

[10] Zubatsky M, Harris SM, Mendenhall TJ. Clinical training and practice patterns of medical family therapists: A national survey. Journal of Marital Family Therapy. 2017;**43**(2):264-275

[11] Szapocznik J et al. Brief strategic family therapy: An intervention to reduce adolescent risk behavior. Journal of Couple Family Psychology: Research Practice. 2012;**1**(2):134

[12] Varghese M, Kirpekar V, Loganathan S. Family interventions: Basic principles and techniques. Journal of Indian Journal of Psychiatry. 2020;**62**(Suppl. 2):S192

[13] Williams-Reade J, Freitas C, Lawson L. Narrative-informed medical family therapy: Using narrative therapy practices in brief medical encounters. Families, Systems, & Health. 2014;**32**:416-425. DOI: 10.1037/fsh0000082

Chapter 2

Innovative Family Therapy for Households in Global Complex Humanitarian Crises

Oluwatoyin Olatundun Ilesanmi, Faith Ibitoyosi Ilesanmi and Raouf Hajji

Abstract

The relief societies are diverse and consist of humanitarian organizations and humanitarian NGOs. They provide emergency aid interventions to victims of armed conflicts, protracted wars, famines, and natural disasters across the globe. The relief societies have witnessed multiple arrays of complex humanitarian catastrophes affecting families in varying degrees in a global dimension and impact. These societies have been providing lifesaving assistance and protection for victims of war, orphans, and vulnerable groups. They have been reducing the impact of humanitarian crises on families and communities, providing aid for recovery and improving preparedness for future emergencies for moral, altruistic, and emotional reasons. Crisis-impacted families may be located far from the fragile locale or in the eye of the storm. Their losses may be psychosocial, economic, or psychological distress or mental health issues. At the onset of the Russian–Ukrainian War, families across the global community are already counting their losses. These call for novel therapeutic interventions among clinicians and counseling psychotherapists. This chapter, therefore, highlights existing strategies for innovative therapeutic measures for families affected by complex humanitarian emergencies.

Keywords: effects, innovative family-focused therapies, households, vulnerable persons, complex humanitarian emergencies

1. Introduction

The humanitarian community is diverse with multiple arrays of complex emergencies (war, natural disasters, famine, armed conflict, food insecurity, climate change, both natural and industrial disasters, and disease outbreaks) with varying severity and impacts on families across the globe [1]. The global community has witnessed waves of violent and protracted complex humanitarian crises in Burkina Faso, Myanmar, Yemen, Venezuela, Ethiopia, Afghanistan, the Democratic Republic of Congo, Nigeria, Iraq, South Sudan, Syria, Somalia, and Ukraine.

Humanitarian catastrophes (conflicts and calamities) pose serious threats to individual families' survival and adaptation [2]. They engender widespread human suffering and destructive events that require a wide range of emergency relief resources and timely intervention.

Although the humanitarian catastrophe-impacted families may be located far from the fragile locale or in the eye of the storm, they may suffer the loss of loved ones, displacement, loss of income, food scarcity, inflation, and the rising cost of living. Accompanying disasters and humanitarian crises are widespread human distress amidst high levels of immediate chaos and delays in the restoration of formal health and social services in the locale of impact [2].

The intensity of the impact of disasters and humanitarian crises such as war, mass conflict, or overwhelming natural disasters on families and households depends on the type, suddenness, and scale of the catastrophe and the socio-cultural and historical context of the domain of occurrence [3]. The over two decades of conflict and political instability and the nascent complex humanitarian crises (Ebola, cholera, COVID-19, and the 2021 volcanic eruption) have worsened the health systems, resulted in high levels of acute food insecurity, and increased the number of internally displaced people (5 million) in the Democratic Republic of Congo (DRC) [2].

In terms of displacement, the UNHCR reported that more than 89.3 million people were classified as forcibly displaced due to conflict, war, violence, persecution, human rights abuses, or events seriously disturbing public order as at the end of 2021 [4, 5]. Part of these displaced persons are 21.3 million refugees under UNHCR's mandate, 5.8 million Palestine refugees under UNRWA's mandate, 53.2 million internally displaced people, 4.6 million asylum seekers, and 4.4 million Venezuelans displaced abroad [5]. The Russian invasion of Ukraine has pushed the figure of forcibly displaced persons to over 100 million [5, 6]. Afghanistan appears to have the largest displaced population globally due to its decades of violent conflict and natural disasters [7].

Families exposed to prolonged and violent conflicts and the Covid-19 pandemic, including displacements, famine, and other forms of humanitarian crises in fragile nations such as Afghanistan, Ethiopia, Myanmar, the central Sahel (Burkina Faso, Mali, and the Niger), Cabo Delgado Province in Mozambique, South Sudan, Sudan, the Bolivarian Republic of Venezuela, and Yemen, suffer losses and severe violations of human dignities, such as torture and sexual violence. The losses usually include psychosocial, economic, or psychological distress (such as anger, depression, grief, etc.) or mental health issues (such as depression, anxiety, post-traumatic stress disorder, psychosis, etc.) [8].

Since the onset of the Russian–Ukrainian War, for instance, families across the global community (Asia, Africa, and global North and South) are already counting their losses [9]. The humanitarian crisis has devastated many families and rendered many stateless and homeless [10]. A lot of the crisis-affected families are currently living under extreme fear and tension; have limited resources to fulfill their needs; live in tents; have limited food, water, and clothing; and face many difficulties and unexpected hardships including cultural and language barrier problems. The refugees' children and international students caught in the war are finding it very hard to continue their education. A lot of such students have had to return to their home country without a clear definitive idea of what the future holds for them [9, 10]. Besides, such families are also experiencing financial difficulties, discrimination, and psychological problems [11, 12].

Among the vulnerable are young couples, children, nursing mothers, and surrogate mothers for international parents, among others. These could be classified as emergency-affected families, veteran families, traumatized and emotionally disturbed families, traumatized couples, suburban couples, single families, non-domiciled/homeless families, aged families, and vulnerable children and orphans.

The impact of complex humanitarian crises on such families is worsened by the emergence of mass destitution, homelessness, statelessness, and mass deportation to their country of origin [13]. This means that they have no home, lack a fixed abode or address, and do not belong to any state. No state considers them as their nationals [14, 15]. These often culminate in an emotional state of feeling lost and deprived of human relationships and increased anxiety [16].

The key psychosocial domains of individual families that are threatened by disasters and humanitarian crises include security and safety; interpersonal bonds and networks (the family, kinship groups, community, and society); identities and roles (parent, worker, student, citizen, social leader, etc.); justice and protection from abuse; and institutions of existential meaning and coherence (traditions, religion, spiritual practices, and political and social participation) [17]. These have great implications on the individual and collective family mental health and well-being.

Article 1 of the United Nations Convention on Status of Refugees stipulated that 'owing to a well-founded fear of being persecuted for reasons of race, religion, nationality, membership of a particular social group, or political opinion', refugees are outside the country of their nationality and are unable to or, owing to such fear, are unwilling to avail themselves of the protection of their host country.

Despite this, there are various universally agreed-upon conventions, declarations, protocols, agreements, laws, and statutes safeguarding and protecting the rights of persons caught in complex humanitarian emergencies including refugees. Examples include the UN Convention Relating to the Status of Refugees, 1951, and Protocol, 1949; Protocol Relating to the Status of Refugees, 1967; the New York Declaration for Refugees and Migrants, 2016; UN Declaration on Territorial Asylum, 1948; Universal Declaration of Human Rights, 1948; Convention Relating to the Status of Stateless Persons, 1954; International Convention on Civil and Political Rights; Convention on the Reduction of Statelessness, 1961; Convention on the Elimination of Discrimination against Women, 1979; and the Guiding Principles on Internal Displacement, 1998. Some of the regional refugee laws are the Cartagena Declaration (1984) and the Asian African Legal Consultative Committee Principles (1996).

The demands of some of these international documents are the need for innovative psychological care of individuals and families vulnerable to disasters and complex humanitarian emergencies. Consequently, the psychological and existential conditions of contemporary persons and families in complex humanitarian emergencies rest principally on Maslow's pyramid of needs—physiological, safety, love, esteem, and self-actualization [18]. Thus, there is an urgent need for novel therapeutic interventions and counseling, especially innovations in family therapy among clinicians and counseling psychotherapists without borders. This chapter, therefore, suggests strategies for innovative therapeutic measures for families affected by complex humanitarian emergencies.

2. Rationale

Sociologically, the family is a major component of society [19]. Healthy families sustain and improve the sociocultural, socioeconomic, and emotional life of healthy societies. In psychological parlance, families are the bedrock and systems of interpersonal interactions for the protection of individual members from societal manipulative influences of society. A family provides individual members with adaptation skills and strategies for proper and effective functioning in life. More so, Vygotsky opines that the family is the most important element of the social situation of an individual's development [20]. However, Shapiro [19] asserts that both the personal and the social are present in disaster-prone and complex humanitarian emergency-ridden terrains.

The impact of complex humanitarian emergencies on families' social situations encompasses a wide range of acute and chronic psychological issues in different settings. It also involves mass displacement of people, homelessness, heightened poverty, and psychosocial problems such as abuse and neglect. These negative effects of disasters and complex humanitarian emergencies on families' social situations sometimes aggravate the different aspects of an individual's existence within the family/household, thereby resulting in the formation of complex personality disorders [21]. Such complexes, psychological problems, crises, and conflicts sometimes require the efforts of family therapy specialists to remedy them [20].

Acknowledging earlier works by the mental health Gap Action Programme Humanitarian Intervention Guide (mhGAP-HIG) [1] on brief versions of structured psychological interventions for people experiencing symptoms of common mental disorders (CMDs), therefore, triggered the need for this paper, which highlights the effects of complex humanitarian crises on families' social situations and the exiting innovative family-focused therapies for households affected by complex humanitarian emergencies in the global community.

3. Research questions

a. What are the varied forms of complex humanitarian emergencies?

b. What are the psychological effects of complex humanitarian crises on families' social situations?

c. What are the exciting innovative family-focused therapies for households affected by complex humanitarian emergencies in the global community?

4. Forms of complex humanitarian emergencies

Complex humanitarian catastrophes (CHC) could be acute crises, cyclical disasters, or man-made complex humanitarian emergencies [22, 23]. Natural disasters such as hurricanes (typhoons), tsunamis, wildfires, tornados, earthquakes, floods, volcanic eruptions, landslides/avalanches, heat waves, and blizzards are examples of acute humanitarian catastrophes [24]. These have been categorized as geophysical disasters such as earthquakes, tsunamis, and volcanic eruptions; hydrological disasters such as floods and avalanches; climatological disasters like droughts; meteorological disasters like storms and cyclones; and biological disasters such as plagues and epidemics.

Examples of cyclical disasters are water insecurity, food insecurity, debilitating/life-threatening endemic diseases, refugee crisis, and internally displaced persons [22]. Man-made complex humanitarian emergencies are forms of disasters triggered by either civil wars or international wars or ethnic cleansing or genocide and resulting in large-scale population displacement with accompanying deterioration of living conditions (such as food, potable water, shelter, and sanitation) and an increase in mortality over a limited period. Examples include the Holocaust in Europe in the 1930s and 1940s, the Bengal Famine of 1943, the murder or expulsion of the Chinese from Indonesia in the 1960s, as well as the more recent wars, ethnic cleansing, forced migration, and genocide occurring in places such as Somalia, Bosnia, Rwanda, Kosovo, Sierra Leone, and East Timor [25].

5. Psychological effects of CHC and Vignettes of innovative therapies

Disasters and humanitarian emergencies are extremely distressing and traumatic events that threaten safety and security, interpersonal bonds, systems of justice, roles and identities, and institutions that promote meaning and coherence [8]. These often take a great toll on people's physical, mental, and psychological well-being, triggering a wide range of emotional, cognitive, behavioral, and somatic reactions among survivors. Some of these wide-ranging effects include:

a. **Fear response:** This is a psychological response (avoidance and arousal responses) to threats of natural or man-made disasters and humanitarian crises. It mobilizes physiological and behavioral reactions that protect individuals from death or injury in the face of violent clashes, wars, genocides, war crimes, etc. As depicted in the vignette below, the intensity of an individual's avoidance and arousal responses to disasters and humanitarian crises could be dynamic, persistent, chronic, and potentially disabling depending on the nature of the crisis [26].

b. **Post-traumatic stress disorders (PTSD)**: These consist of psychological issues (re-experiencing, avoidance, and a heightened sense of current threat) resulting from exposure to any form of natural or complex humanitarian crisis.

Vignette of constant fear of insecurity and fear of the worst in the voice of a young mother, who suddenly became the head of her home in Southern Kaduna, Nigeria

Hadiza, a petty trader and young mother of four (one girl and three boys), widowed when armed bandits raided Hayin Kanwa village, Yakawada ward in Giwa Local Government Area of Kaduna State, Nigeria, sat amidst the children on a badly tattered mat in the cool of the day sharing a meal of "tuwo" in front of their small mud brick home, made up of two rooms. While the children devoured the meal prepared by their mother, suddenly, Hadiza lost in thoughts and with a sobered burdened face, filled with worries, gazed into the distance, and pondering how she will sustain her four children: 8, 6, 4, and 2 years of age.

When asked, "why are you not eating with the children?" She responded, "I am in deep pain." Hadiza sobbed and then stated further, "The children and I survived unknown gunmen attacks by mere luck." Her husband was killed for delaying opening the door of their home to the bandits when they attacked the community. "I feel helpless, without my husband I do not know how I will cope; paying for food every day, paying school fees and buying medicines when the children fall sick, it is a big responsibility that troubles me. Besides, I do not know how I can protect my sons from being kidnapped by the bandits and my daughter from being raped if the bandits attacked again."

The loss of Hadiza's husband to bandits' attacks deepened her poverty status and plunged her into sadness, sorrow, and persistent grief. The children, who are oblivious to the depth of their mother's pain, are likely to experience further traumatic encounters with the unknown bandits, who have persistently been shooting people and burning houses including religious buildings in rural communities across the state.

Psychologists attending to young poor widows like Hadiza, who can be diagnosed with manifesting co-occurring post-traumatic depression and anxiety, need to deploy hands-on skills for resilience and hope-building. Although Nigerian psychologists are not trained as humanitarian actors, to fit into this mode, there is the need for them to acquire psychotherapeutic and counseling skills necessary for trauma counseling in highly volatile and disaster crisis-prone settings like Northern Nigeria. Such skill sets will include resilience building (the ability to rebound, bounce back, and overcome), assessment skills necessary for uncovering and disrupting negative automatic thoughts, and listening skills.

a. **Acute traumatic stress disorders**: Acute traumatic stress disorder may be a normative response to disasters and humanitarian crises. It often tends to subside once conditions of safety are established. Symptoms include a wide range of non-specific psychological and medically unexplained physical complaints.

b. **Insomnia and other sleep problems:** Insomnia with considerable difficulty in daily functioning is one of the problems commonly experienced by individuals after experiencing extreme stress due to exposure to any form of natural or complex humanitarian crisis. Psychologically oriented interventions (e.g., relaxation techniques) may be considered for any family experiencing insomnia.

Vignette of Transient mental trauma and sleep disturbances experienced by a father and two sons in East Nusa Tenggara islands in 2021

John, a father of two, who lost his wife to the deadly Indonesian cyclone Seroja in the East Nusa Tenggara islands, reported that his children experienced temporary mental trauma and sleep disturbances, which is manifested by crying when a sudden change in the weather occurs. The cyclone brought strong winds and heavy rains that triggered flash floods and landslides. "I cry every time the wind becomes stronger. (I cry) because I recall (the event)." I do not want the typhoon to recur in their place. I do not want my children and me to be killed. The cyclone resulted in a complicated tragedy and sadness. I cannot sleep for a day."

Sleep disturbances are often referred to as a hallmark and core symptom of PTSD. The literature affirms that untreated sleep disturbances can worsen the exacerbation of PTSD symptoms, which may have negative effects on a patient's treatment response and constitute a risk factor for poor treatment outcomes. The mental health treatment as usual (TAU) for PTSD comprises 10 sessions with a medical doctor (pharmacological treatment and psychoeducation) and 16–20 sessions with a psychologist (manual-based cognitive behavioral therapy) for a period of 8 to 12 months.

Bruhn, Laugesen, Kromann-Larsen, Trevino, Eplov, Hjorthøj, and Carlsson's [27] utilization of add-on (integrated care) intervention to TAU strengthened the coordination between mental health treatment and employment interventions with three cross-sectoral collaborative meetings during the mental health treatment. It drew attention to the bidirectional impact of mental health problems and post-migration stressors and focused on cross-sectoral shared plans.

The primary outcome is functioning, measured by WHODAS 2.0, the interviewer-administered 12-item version, with secondary outcomes measuring the quality of life, mental health symptoms, and post-migration stressors.

In another study, Sandahl and Jennum [28] utilized add-on treatment with mianserin and/or Imagery Rehearsal Therapy (IRT) in addition to TAU as a sleep-enhancing treatment in refugees (18 years or older) with PTSD at a Danish outpatient clinic. The refugees were from Afghanistan, Ex-Yugoslavia, Iraq, Iran, Lebanon, and Syria. The TAU was an interdisciplinary treatment approach covering a period of 6–8 months with pharmacological treatment, physiotherapy, psychoeducation, and manual-based cognitive behavioral therapy within a framework of weekly sessions with a physician, physiotherapist, or psychologist.

a. **Somatoform disorders**: These are psychological thoughts, feelings, and behaviors such as constant worry and fear about potential illness or signs of severe physical illness even when there is no evidence as a result of exposure to natural disasters such as chemical weapons and other forms of complex humanitarian crises.

b. **Complicated/prolonged grief disorder**: Grief is the emotional suffering people feel after a loss of homes and livelihoods or bereavement due to any form of natural or complex humanitarian crisis. This emotional reaction may be self-limiting without becoming a mental disorder or may prolong over an extended period. Prolonged grief disorder involves a severe preoccupation with or intense longing for the deceased person accompanied by intense emotional pain and considerable difficulty with daily functioning for at least 6 months (and for a period that is much longer than what is expected in the person's culture). Symptoms of prolonged grief disorder include moderate–severe depressive disorder (DEP), psychosis (PSY), harmful use of alcohol and drugs (SUB), self-harm/suicide (SUI), and other significant mental health complaints (OTH).

c. **Depression/helplessness**: This may range from moderate to severe depressive disorder (DEP) for individuals or among family members who have been exposed to any form of natural or complex humanitarian crisis.

Vignette of Catastrophizing/Reminiscence, Selflessness, Bonding, and Rebuilding Lives

The overall intensity and catastrophe of 2013 super typhoon Haiyan (locally known as Yolanda), which hit the town of Visayas, the northern part of Cebu, Philippines on November 8, 2013, left families and all its victims (children to the older population) living with a deep sense of helplessness, intense fear, confusing, and sometimes frightening emotional toll [29]

The devastation impaired the sensory awareness and physical mobility of many. It also worsened their health conditions and weakened their social and economic capabilities. The survivors experienced fear, difficulty, loss, helplessness before and during the typhoon, and sadness by the loss of the properties they had invested in for many years due to the calamity. The typhoon-induced aggravated fear including fear of personal safety, security of loved ones, the absence of mature family members who can help protect them in the family, and fear of death at the height of the catastrophe.

In Visayas, the less affected young and older adults looked out for their neighbors, supported distressed families, mobilized resources, and cared for orphans and vulnerable children (OVC) and other dependents during the traumatic event. After the crisis, they were able to reminisce about their experience and rebuild their lives and community.

The survivors in the Visayas compensated for their feelings of intense fear, loss, and helplessness, with a sense of selflessness, strengthening social bonds, rebuilding their lives, and reminiscence. Through reminiscence, they tried reliving memories and compared them with their current experiences. Sharing memories helps older adults to relive and explore their thoughts and feelings about their unique traumatic experience of the typhoon. They were also able to put their past experiences in perspective with what is happening to them in the present or what is expected to happen in the future. Thus, reminiscence, social bonding, and rebuilding became the mechanism for coping with changes in their life situation or circumstances. Sales and Pinazo-Hernandis [30] opine that reminiscence therapy (consisting of 10 sessions lasting 60 min each) is a psychological intervention that can be used to assist an individual to remember and interpret life events, feelings, and thoughts that define and give meaning to him/her. Reminiscence of earlier emergency experiences, coping strategies, traditional skills, and local environmental knowledge can result in positive mental health for survivors of catastrophic emergencies.

a. **Psychosis (PSY)**: The symptoms include abnormal behavior (e.g., strange appearance, self-neglect, incoherent speech, wandering, mumbling, or laughing to self), strange beliefs, hearing voices or seeing things that are not there, extreme suspicion, lack of desire to be with or talk with others, and lack of motivation to do daily chores and work.

Vignette for refugees with a high burden of unaddressed grief, loss, trauma, and depression

Assefa, a refugee who fled from the conflict in Tigray to Gedaref, a state in eastern Sudan with his family, recounted how his family had struggled to support his daughter, who was experiencing a mental health condition: "Almaz is my daughter. The situation in Tigray affected her mental health and she started behaving violently and erratically. We did not know how to manage things, so we used to tie her up. I tied her up in our car on our way here, tied her up in the tent we were given, and later at our house. There was no health facility available at the time, nor any medication for her treatment."

Besides Assefa's case, Pieter Ventevogel, a senior mental health and psychosocial support officer with UNHCR, reported the high burden of unaddressed grief, loss, trauma, and depression among refugees, who fled from Tigray, Ethiopia, to eastern Sudan in 2022. He also reported cases of unaddressed gender-based violence among female refugees and saw children depicting violence and dead bodies in their drawings.

a. **Survivors of sexual and gender-based violence (S/GBV)**: Incidences of sexual and gender-based violence in conflict settings are risk factors for mental health and psychosocial well-being. The World Report on Violence and Health posits that these are any form of sexual act, attempted sexual act, unwanted sexual comments or advances, acts of human trafficking, or otherwise directed against any person's sexuality through coercive means regardless of their relationship in any setting [31]. All women, girls, boys, men, and unaccompanied minors, who have been vulnerable to such violent abuses in conflict-affected settings and during forced displacement, should be offered trauma-focused cognitive processing family therapy [32].

b. **Social avoidance/social withdrawal**: Any survivor of a complex humanitarian crisis exhibiting social avoidance also needs family therapies.

c. **Irritability and aggressive behavior**: Teenagers who have been exposed to or witnessed complex humanitarian crises tend to act irritably and repeat abusive behaviors—fight, engage in risky sexual activities, or dabble in drugs and alcohol.

d. **Harmful use of alcohol and drugs (SUB)**: Humanitarian crisis can worsen the harmful use of alcohol, narcotic drug use, and air pollution. The SDG Target 3.5 on mental health aims at strengthening the prevention and treatment of substance abuse, including narcotic drug abuse and harmful use of alcohol. Consequently, family psychotherapists need to be able to manage harmful use of alcohol and drugs as well as life-threatening withdrawal among anyone affected by a humanitarian crisis.

e. **Suicide (SUI) and suicidal risks**: Suicidal behavior (suicide attempt, suicide, and suicidal ideation) can be triggered by traumatic experiences of hazardous journeys, the loss of resources and belongings, death of loved ones, separation from family members, harsh circumstances in refugee camps, and direct exposure to armed conflict and violence, war, and torture [33].

6. The psychological needs of families affected by humanitarian crises

Exposure to disasters and complex humanitarian crises such as genocide,

Based on Abraham Maslow's [34] hierarchy of needs, the following are the basic needs of family members and whole families caught up with and directly impacted by humanitarian crises:

1. **Physiological Needs:** Physiological needs are the basic needs and requirements for the body to survive—water, clean air (oxygen), food, and sleep. These are the basic needs of anyone caught up in a humanitarian crisis.

2. **Security Needs**: Security needs include the need for a safe family environment, steady employment, a safe neighborhood, and a stable financial situation.

3. **Social Needs:** Social needs include the need for belonging, love, intimacy, and affection. Relationships with friends, romantic partners, and families fulfill this need, as does involvement in communities and social or religious groups.

4. **Esteem Needs**: Esteem needs include the need for validation from others (status, respect, recognition, and reputation) and positive self-evaluation (competence, confidence in ability, accomplishment, and skills mastery).

5. **Self-Actualization Needs**: This category includes the need to maximize one's potential or the need for personal growth, creativity, morality, and meaning making.

7. Innovative psychosocial support and family-focused therapies for groups and households affected by complex humanitarian emergencies

The following are the psychosocial support and family-focused therapies that should be deployed for treating psychological distress and strengthening the mental health and well-being of adolescents, families, kinship groups, orphans and vulnerable groups, unaccompanied children, and communities in humanitarian settings:

a. **Psychosocial Supports**: Psychosocial support programs address the emotional, social, mental, and spiritual needs of persons and families in crisis. They help in building resilience in children and families. They essentially focus on people's experiences of humanitarian crises within broader social dimensions to facilitate individual and community resilience strategies to mitigate that impact. They can be provided at the individual, family, and community levels by promoting and providing everyday activities such as schooling, activating social networks, as well as developing and building on existing coping mechanisms to manage the impact of humanitarian crises.

   For unaccompanied children, orphans, and vulnerable children in humanitarian settings, the main goal of psychosocial support programs is to ensure that they are properly placed in stable and supportive family environments. They also focus on how family members respond to the harsh realities of humanitarian catastrophes based on their age, gender, and circumstances.

   The following are some of the basic psychosocial support programs recommended for individuals or families experiencing serious psychosocial and emotional distress due to their exposure to complex humanitarian emergencies:

   i. **Psychological first aid (PFA)**: PFA is needed immediately after the occurrence of an extremely stressful event. It begins with the identification of the current psychosocial stressors experienced by and the basic needs of all or any members of the family through stress management techniques such as listening to their unpressurized communication and probing for their psychosocial needs and concerns. PFA strategies for addressing their current psychosocial stressors entail the reactivation and strengthening of their family social support networks by providing direct or indirect psychosocial support through socialization processes such as family gatherings, visit to neighbors, and participation in community activities. They also entail the provision of access to services and protection from further harm. The greatest need of families affected by disasters and humanitarian emergencies is to be heard or listened to.

   ii. **Psychoeducation programs**: This entails training on stress management and normal reactions to grief and acute stress. These programs solely provide education on the impact of exposure to humanitarian crises and seek to empower people by promoting awareness and managing the impact of that exposure via educational materials and tools.

   iii. **Health-related interventions**: During humanitarian crises, psychosocial support activities can be integrated into existing community and health systems and can foster support groups for parents, families, community caregivers, and youth (peers).

b. **Family-focused therapies:** Family-focused counseling and psychotherapies are the mainstays of intervention treatment for mental disorders [35]. Highlighted below are some of the effective family therapies that could be used for households affected by complex humanitarian emergencies:

i. **Problem-solving psychotherapy:** This is a cognitive–behavioral intervention geared toward improving an individual's ability to cope with stressful life experiences. It can be utilized with vulnerable groups and families during humanitarian emergencies based on the assumption that symptoms of psychopathology may be a negative consequence of maladaptive adjustment and coping to the crisis events. Examples of these modes of intervention include psychoeducation, interactive problem-solving exercises, and motivational homework assignments [36].

ii. **Interpersonal therapy (IPT):** This is a benchmark therapy for depression and other mental health conditions that are elevated in humanitarian settings. Administering interpersonal therapy (IPT) as a family-focused therapy should be the first-line treatment for pregnant and breastfeeding women, survivors of gender-based violence, and families mourning the loss of their loved ones in humanitarian settings.

iii. **Behavioral activation therapy:** This action-oriented approach is a structured treatment suited for use among individuals with co-occurring depression and substance use disorders (SUDs). It reduces the symptoms of depression and substance dependence through the activation of increasing rewarding experiences in their lives. Scheduling of the behavioral activation activities and other techniques to be completed outside the brief manualized therapy sessions should be done collaboratively by the therapists and individual vulnerable groups/families exposed to humanitarian crises.

iv. **Relaxation techniques:** Autogenic training, deep breathing, progressive muscle relaxation, massage, tai chi, yoga, biofeedback, music and art therapy, aromatherapy, meditation, and guided imagery can be used to move distressed people in humanitarian settings into a deep state of relaxation [37].

v. **Gestalt family therapy**: This provides face-to-face talk or body psychotherapy and addresses the intrapsychic and interpersonal impact of humanitarian crises to support improved overall psychological functioning and coping skills.

vi. **Cognitive behavioral therapy (CBT)**: CBT provides face-to-face, individual, or group-talking therapy (i.e., not online or via media or other materials) as well as a digital or Internet-delivered mode of intervention. It is useful in exploring and making explicit links between specific thoughts, emotions, somatic and non-somatic feelings, and behaviors of families within and outside the terrains of complex humanitarian crises. It is effective in positively changing a person's thinking ('cognitive') to elicit change in what they do (behavioral) [38]. Digital or Internet-delivered cognitive behavioral therapy (iCBT) is a short-term therapist-assisted Internet-delivered therapeutic intervention for improving the well-being and overall mental health of families in complex humanitarian emergencies. The treatment program components consist of eight text-based modules, where each module is expected to be completed within 1 week.

vii. **Narrative exposure therapy (NET)**: This exposure-based, psychodynamic, narrative, and supportive counseling therapy is useful for the reduction of PTSD, depression, stress, and anxiety symptoms as well as improvement of functioning among individuals and families affected by humanitarian crises [39]. It was effectively used for the psychosocial management of refugees in Uganda [40], the survivors of the 2008 Sichuan earthquake in China [41], Mozambican civil war survivors [42], and widowed and orphaned survivors of the Rwandan genocide [43]. NET can be used to facilitate exposure to specific or non-specific reminders, cues, or memories related to exposure to a traumatic event [38]. It can be used to help persons or families affected by complex humanitarian emergencies to reconstruct a consistent and/or coherent narrative about their traumatic experience either verbally or through writing to aid symptom reduction [38]. Examples of NET include:

- **Brief testimony psychotherapy**: This short-term therapy is useful for the psychosocial treatment of traumatized victims of war or other organized violence. The therapy consists of 12 sessions that enable patients to narrate their life stories, including traumatic experiences [44]. This brief therapy consists of six sessions, of approximately 90 minutes, weekly or biweekly [39].

8. Conclusion

Mitigating emergencies is necessary to overcome the overwhelming burden of losses faced by communities in distress. This paper looked into the psychological effects of complex humanitarian crises on families, the psychological needs of families affected by humanitarian crises, and therapies for groups and households affected by complex humanitarian emergencies. Therefore, this chapter emphasizes the need for innovative psychosocial support and family-focused therapies in the management of complex humanitarian crises.

Author details

Oluwatoyin Olatundun Ilesanmi[1]*, Faith Ibitoyosi Ilesanmi[2] and Raouf Hajji[3]

1 Centre for Gender and Humanitarian and Development Studies, Redeemer's University, Ede, Nigeria

2 Centre for Gender, Health and Social Rehabilitation, Ile-Ife, Nigeria

3 Internal Medicine Department, Sidi Bouzid Hospital, Medicine Faculty of Sousse, University of Sousse, Tunisia

*Address all correspondence to: ilesanmit@run.edu.ng

References

[1] World Health Organization and United Nations High Commissioner for Refugees. mhGAP Humanitarian Intervention Guide (mhGAP-HIG): Clinical management of mental, neurological and substance use conditions in humanitarian emergencies. Geneva: WHO; 2015

[2] Claude KM, Serge MS, Alexis KK, Hawkes MT. Prevention of COVID-19 in internally displaced persons camps in War-Torn North Kivu, Democratic Republic of the Congo: A mixed-methods study. Global Health: Science and Practice. 2020;**8**(4):638-653

[3] Porter M, Haslam N. Predisplacement and Postdisplacement Factors Associated With Mental Health of Refugees and Internally Displaced Persons: A Meta-analysis. JAMA. 2005;**294**(5):602-612. DOI:10.1001/jama.294.5.602

[4] Heisey J, Sánchez IA, Bernagros A. Working for Inclusion: Economic Inclusion in Contexts of Forced Displacement. PEI In Practice; Vol.4. Washington, DC: © World Bank; 2022. http://localhost:4000//entities/publication/525fefe2-7e77-5607-ba9c-5b3cf2917bc8 License: CC BY 3.0 IGO

[5] UNHCR. Global Trends: Forced Displacement in 2020. UNHCR; 2021. Statistics and Demographics Section UNHCR Global Data Service UN City, Marmorvej 51 2100 Copenhagen, Denmark. stats@unhcr.org

[6] Legg SJI. Displaced people: Tragedy and triumph?: The case of Ukraine. Interaction. 2022;**50**(2):23-25. DOI: 10.3316/informit.511618457243973

[7] Sasse G. War and displacement: The case of Ukraine. Journal of Europe-Asia Studies. 2020;**72**(3):347-353

[8] Silove D, Steel Z. Understanding community psychosocial needs after disasters: Implications for mental health services. Psychology, Medicine Journal of Postgraduate Medicine. 2006; **52**(2):121

[9] Armitage R. War in Ukraine: the impacts on child health. Journal of British Journal of General Practice. 2022; **72**(719):272-273

[10] Vus V, Esterlis I. Support of the population within the Russian-Ukrainian war: Insider's perspective. Journal of Chronic Stress. 2022;**6**: 24705470221101884

[11] Chaaya C et al. Ukraine–Russia crisis and its impacts on the mental health of Ukrainian young people during the COVID-19 pandemic. Journal of Annals of Medicine Surgery. 2022;**79**:104033

[12] Mbah RE, Wasum DF. Russian-Ukraine 2022 war: A review of the economic impact of Russian-Ukraine crisis on the USA, UK, Canada, and Europe. Journal of Advances in Social Sciences Research Journal. 2022;**9**(3):144-153

[13] Siegelberg ML. Statelessness: A modern history. United State of America: Harvard University Press; 2020

[14] Eliassi B. Homelessness and statelessness: Possibilities and perils. In: Cohen R, Fischer C, editors. Routledge Handbook of Diaspora Studies. Routledge; 2018. pp. 120-128. ProQuest Ebook Central, http://ebookcentral.proquest.com/lib/linne-ebooks/detail.action?docID=5580215

[15] Siddika BA. Impact of statelessness: Are we ready to face? Journal of Open Journal of Social Sciences. 2019;**7**(12):1-11

[16] Colonnello P. Chapter 6 Homelessness as Heimatlosigkeit?. In: The Ethics of Homelessness. Leiden, The Netherlands: Brill; 2020. DOI: 10.1163/9789004420366_008

[17] Copolov C, Knowles A. An exploration of the adaptation and development after persecution (ADAPT) model with young adult Hazaras from refugee backgrounds in Australia. Journal of Transcultural Psychiatry. 2021;**58**(2):187-199

[18] Desmet P, Fokkinga S. Interaction, Beyond Maslow's pyramid: Introducing a typology of thirteen fundamental needs for human-centered design. Journal of Multimodal Technologies. 2020;**4**(3):38

[19] Shapiro AZ. The concept of positivity in family therapy and the task of psychological assistance to the contemporary Russian family. Journal of Russian East European Psychology. 1997; **35**(6):73-92

[20] Vygotsky L, Cole M. Lev Vygotsky: Learning and social constructivism. Learning theories for early years practice, 66, 58. MacBlain, Sean - London: SAGE Publications Ltd; 2018. p. 120. ISBN: 9781526450753. Permalink: http://digital.casalini.it/9781526450753. Casalini id: 5018183

[21] Jung CG, de Laszlo, Violet S. The Basic Writings of C.G. Jung: Revised Edition, Princeton: Princeton University Press; 1991. DOI: 10.1515/9780691229782

[22] Iserson KV. Tackling the global challenge: Humanitarian catastrophes. Journal of Western Journal of Emergency Medicine. 2014;**15**(2):231

[23] O'Keefe M. Chronic crises in the arc of insecurity: A case study of Karamoja. Journal of Third World Quarterly. 2010; **31**(8):1271-1295

[24] Horn S, Reinhart CM, Trebesch C. Coping with Disasters: Two Centuries of International Official Lending. Policy Research Working Paper;No. 9612. © World Bank, Washington, DC. 2021. http://localhost:4000//entities/publication/9a50e81e-6f94-5406-929d-d9f37c1fba8f License: CC BY 3.0 IGO

[25] National Research Council (US) Roundtable on the Demography of Forced Migration. In: Reed HE, Keely CB, editors. Forced Migration & Mortality. Washington (DC): National Academies Press (US); 2001. 3, Famine, Mortality, and Migration: A Study of North Korean Migrants in China. Available from: https://www.ncbi.nlm.nih.gov/books/NBK223341/

[26] Steel Z et al. Impact of immigration detention and temporary protection on the mental health of refugees. Journal of the British Journal of Psychiatry. 2006; **188**(1):58-64

[27] Bruhn M et al. The effect of an integrated care intervention of multidisciplinary mental health treatment and employment services for trauma-affected refugees: Study protocol for a randomised controlled trial. Journal of Clinical Trials. 2022;**23**(1):859

[28] Sandahl H et al. Treatment of sleep disturbances in trauma-affected refugees: Study protocol for a randomised controlled trial. Journal of Clinical Trails. 2017;**18**:1-13

[29] Johnson H, Ling C, McBee E. Multi-disciplinary Care for the Elderly in Disasters: An Integrative Review. Prehospital and Disaster Medicine. 2015; **30**(1):72-79. DOI:10.1017/S1049023X14001241

[30] Sales A, Pinazo-Hernandis S, Martinez D. Effects of a reminiscence program on meaning of life, sense of

coherence and coping in older women living in nursing homes during COVID-19. In Healthcare. 2022;**10**(2):188. MDPI

[31] Krug EG, Mercy JA, Dahlberg LL, Zwi AB. The world report on violence and health. The lancet. 2002;**360**(9339): 1083-1088

[32] Ryan GK et al. Lay-delivered talk therapies for adults affected by humanitarian crises in low-and middle-income countries. Journal of Conflict and Health. 2021;**15**(1):1-16

[33] Tinghög P. Migration, Stress and Mental Ill Health: Post-migration Factors and Experiences in the Swedish Context (PhD dissertation, Linköping University Electronic Press). Linköping Studies in Arts and Science No. 480. Dissertations on Health and Society No. 16. Linköping: Department of Medical and Health Sciences, Linköping University Electronic Press, Linköping University; 2009

[34] Maslow AH. A Dynamic Theory of Human Motivation. In: Stacey CL, DeMartino M, editors. Understanding human motivation. Howard Allen Publishers. 1958. pp. 26-47. DOI: 10.1037/11305-004

[35] Silove D, Ventevogel P, Rees S. The contemporary refugee crisis: An overview of mental health challenges. Journal of World Psychiatry. 2017;**16**(2): 130-139

[36] D'Zurilla TJ, Nezu AM. Problem-solving therapy. Journal of Handbook of Cognitive-Behavioral Therapies. 2010;**3**: 197-225

[37] Norelli SK, Long A, Krepps JM. Relaxation Techniques. In: StatPearls. Treasure Island (FL): StatPearls Publishing; 2022. PMID: 30020610

[38] Bangpan M, Felix L, Dickson K. Mental health and psychosocial support programmes for adults in humanitarian emergencies: A systematic review and meta-analysis in low and middle-income countries. British Medical Journal Global Health. 2019;**4**(5):e001484

[39] Weine SM et al. Testimony psychotherapy in Bosnian refugees: A pilot study. American Journal of Psychiatry. 1998;**155**(12):1720-1726

[40] Neuner F et al. A comparison of narrative exposure therapy, supportive counseling, and psychoeducation for treating posttraumatic stress disorder in an African refugee settlement. Journal of Consulting Clinical Psychology. 2004; **72**(4):579

[41] Zang Y, Hunt N, Cox T. A randomised controlled pilot study: The effectiveness of narrative exposure therapy with adult survivors of the Sichuan earthquake. BMC Psychiatry. 2013;**13**(1):1-11. DOI: 10.1186/1471-244X-13-41

[42] Igreja V et al. Testimony method to ameliorate post-traumatic stress symptoms: Community-based intervention study with Mozambican civil war survivors. The British Journal of Psychiatry. 2004;**184**(3):251-257

[43] Jacob N et al. Dissemination of psychotherapy for trauma spectrum disorders in postconflict settings: A randomized controlled trial in Rwanda. Journal of Psychosomatics Psychotherapy. 2014;**83**(6):354-363

[44] van Dijk JA, Schoutrop MJ, Spinhoven P. Testimony therapy: Treatment method for traumatized victims of organized violence. American Journal of Psychotherapy. 2003;**57**(3): 361-373

Chapter 3

Perspective Chapter: Theoretical Paradigm for Mental Health and Family Therapy within the South African Context – An Overview

Barry Lachlan Kevin Viljoen

Abstract

This chapter places focus on family therapy within the African and more specifically South African context. It attempts to sketch a context on a continental level, highlighting and describing the theoretical paradigm through which contextually appropriate theory and literature is being developed. A brief overview is given of mental health within the content. A more specific South African context is then described. Whilst also engaging with limitations and obstacles, also highlighting developments within the context.

Keywords: family therapy, African-centred paradigm, African context, interactional pattern analysis, mental health

1. Introduction

This Chapter will focus on my personal clinical experience, exposure and training in family therapy, within the South African context. This having been in both the private and state sector, from a primary to tertiary level of healthcare. However, with this contextual limitation kept in mind, considering that Africa is a continent, made up of 54 countries, and that diversity will exist on geographical, political, economic levels of resource and perhaps most importantly culturally. It is within these limitations I will attempt to sketch the current landscape of family therapy within the continent.

Whilst having highlighted the disparities which exist, there are also similarities, embraced in the concept of Pan African Humanness. This concept argues that there exists a greater level of commonality amongst the people of Africa, as opposed to the differences [1]. It is through the use of this concept that a theoretical framework has come to be, in which cultural and intellectual developments have taken place [1, 2]. As a result, we have seen the developed and subsequent rise of an African-centred paradigm, which has allowed for Africans to not only have been given a voice, but allowed for that voice to be heard, with regards to life experiences, ancestry, history and tradition [1, 2].

In response to this, the chapter will initially expand upon the African paradigm, setting the context with regards to culture and worldview of Africa. An attempt will then be made to sketch the landscape of mental health within this context. Finally, there will be a specific focus on systemic family therapy within this context, examining the challenges and developments within the field.

2. African epistemology

Western Cultures hold the underlying assumption that humans are innately flawed, with challenges of self-control, manifesting itself in phenomena such as "original sin", which will guide us in the direction of these impulses [3]. However, within African beliefs people are born innately good, and that through interpersonal relationships, they are able to develop their humanness, in a constructive and positive manner [4]. In this regard, being a good member of your community is of greater value as opposed to the accumulation of goods or wealth [5]. The inverse is possible, should actions be viewed as not in keeping with the interests of community, and rather self-serving in nature, they can be viewed as the cause of pain and or misery for others [6]. For this reason, it is argued that African morality is relational [4].

Whilst there is an obvious pluralism and diversity within cultural experience and history, across the continent, it is argued that there is a metaphysical unity and central worldview which exists amongst all Africans [7]. This is highlighted in the stance that nothing is absolute and that the relationship between the natural and supernatural order is governed by the principal of complementary opposites [7].

The Afrocentric paradigm refers to the ideology and the epistemology through which contemporary African-centred practice is rooted, so as for the worldview of Africans, as well as the philosophical assumptions, which are underpinning this, to be acknowledged and given voice [8]. Grounded within African epistemological reflections would be the mindset of commonality and centredness, which builds the frame of the process of knowing within this context [1].

The African context places focus on a collectivistic orientation as opposed to individualistic one [5]. This is thought to be a corner of African thought and life. From this perspective it assumes that everyone belongs and that there is no-one who does not belong [9]. Here the individual is not of lesser importance than the group [5]. As such it can be argued that neither is placed in a hierarchal order. Thus, a person remains a person regardless of their status in life and that their value as a human being is seen to be just as important as another person [9]. The manner in which an individual obtains their own good, is through the good of the group [5].

One such concept to have emerged from this paradigm is the concept of "botho /ubuntu". This concept of "botho /ubuntu", is South African of origin, and has attracted significant attention within several fields. It has usually been described in terms of values, respect, compassion, humility, which are believed to have been rooted within culture, which are collectivist in nature [10]. This concept is considered to have been made up of four key elements, these being African spirituality, personhood, interconnectedness and communalism [10]. These values are thought to be innate to all human beings [5].

African reality has been described as having been made up by three hierarchical, interrelated and not oppositional worlds. These are the microcosmos, which is made up of the immediate perceptible world; the mesocosms which has been made up of the intermediate world of spirits, which are beneficial or malevolent in nature; the third realm is that of the Devine or macrocosmos which is made up of ancestors and spirit beings [1]. Thus, it is believed that within the African structure there is a constant interactional relationship between those who dwell within, these realms and the realms of reality themselves [1].

How do these realms interact and engage? Ancestors operate as a conduit, between the living and God, allowing for communication to take place [10]. Traditional healers are believed to possess the abilities to engage with the spiritual world, able to communicate with the ancestors. As a result, they are often highly regarded members of their respective communities [10]. Within the African context, when a person experiences troubles and or challenges within their life, spiritual healers are often the first port or call. The purpose of which is to establish the nodal cause of the challenge, which is done through their spiritual powers [10].

It is believed that spiritual relationship between the living and ancestors, is not only vertical but also horizontal [11]. What this means is that the quality relationships amongst people as well as their relationship with God and the ancestors will impact upon their personhood.

Mental illness within the Afrocentric paradigm, is rooted within the African cultural and worldview that there are interconnected worlds which influence one another. In this regard it can emanate from any of the realms previously described. For this reason, those who are able to communicate with spiritual forces are often employed, so as to determine the root cause and the intention with which those have become ill [8].

3. Psychopathology from this paradigm

Taking into mind the cultural formulation which has been outlined. One can understand the cultural barriers which exist and limit, if not dissuade individuals from seeking treatment for mental health conditions, from mental health care practitioners, trained in Western-based medicine. For this reason, this stigma or fear needs to be understood [12]. This as it could also be considered a cause for the defaulting of treatment [12]. An example of this, was highlighted in a study conducted in Nigeria, where it was frequently believed that mental illness was a result of moral failing or wickedness [12].

It can and has been argued that the manner in which psychopathology is constructed and understood, and as a result approached in a vastly different manner within Afrocentric and Eurocentric paradigms [8]. For this reason, greater value is often placed in consultation with alternative healthcare providers, such as faith healer and indigenous healers, as opposed to consultation with medical health professionals [13]. Consultations occurring across varying health systems, can be complex, due to the epistemological foundations are quite different which can make collaborative engagements quite challenging [13]. However, this should be effectively managed that it can yield very positive and beneficial outcomes.

In order to achieve this level of collaboration, it would be considered to be of value to understand psychopathology through an African lens. From an African perspective, psychopathology is viewed as an aspect of social drama, which can be experienced as two kinds of dramatic experience, social drama and stage dramas [14]. Social drama can be understood as a breach, from which a crisis develops and requires a remedial process or redress intervention [14]. Whilst stage dramas are socially based, with the aim being to depict approaches which can be engaged with to overcome real social dramas of existence, which can then be effectively overcome [14]. Thus, psychopathology can be seen as a breach in the normal routine of a person's existence, which their inner and outer equilibrium, move towards illness and distress, as opposed to that of harmony and peace [8]. It is believed that ancestors have the ability to grant rewards to the living, whilst also in cases can insight bad luck or illness if unappeased [10].

It is important to hold this formulation in mind. When western psychiatric perspectives have been administered, and have not resulted in a curative response, in which there has been a complete resolution of illness and or symptomatology. The challenge can be that there is an assumption from an Afrocentric paradigm that a hidden message is carried by the illness, which is required to be understood, before a curative intervention can be implemented [8]. It is important to then shift focus to who is speaking through the illness and then the next aspect would be what is expected to be done, so as for a resolution to take place [8]. As such psychological illnesses can be approached as meta-communications, which are rather to be interpreted or "read" as opposed to classified and categorised, as is the case in the Diagnostic and Statistical Manual of Mental Disorders 5 (DSM5) [8]. For this reason, if the two views are held as mutually exclusive, it may result in greater levels of non-adherence to western medical interventions. Allowing for the two to coexist, allowing for greater levels of autonomy and a more active engagement in the treatment process [15].

The value and positive impact of social relationships, on both physical and mental health have been well documented in the context of the global north [16, 17]. Within the African context, this has the added benefit of social capital [18]. Whilst also having cultural significance, specifically within collectivist cultures, which are rooted in the interconnected nature of people [18]. For this reason, it is argued that in order to understand the African episteme, all of these realms must be considered [1].

4. Mental health within the African context

It is believed that mental health is an essential aspect of human health, however if we are to achieve humane and effective treatment of mental health conditions there needs to be an increase in the social, financial and human resources allocated to it [19].

Currently it is estimated that mental health disorders account for 37% of healthy life years lost through disease [12]. Global data suggests that in low to middle income countries that there are insufficient resources, along with an inequity of distribution of these resources [19]. For example, there is only one neuro-psychiatric hospital within the Niger Delta of Nigeria, which services a population of over four million [12]. As such it is estimated that less than 20% of persons with mental illness are able to receive treatment within Nigeria [12].

The current stance is that a balance between hospital-based and community-based services would be the most effective means of provision of mental healthcare [19]. Though this only appears to be the reality within a few of the high-income countries on the continent, with the provision of mental health services outside of the hospital setting only being available in about half of African countries [19]. Patterns of consultation are thought to vary depending on cultural groups and the types of services available or accessible [13].

It is important to note that political instability and general unrest have negatively impacted upon access to as well as the availability of mental healthcare services. The result, a fairly obvious one, is that in areas of conflict, more especially those in which are regularly occurring or frequent, there is a notable absence of mental healthcare professionals [20]. Even though these services are most likely to be more crucially required, as a result of the political and historical context.

Currently we are faced with a lack of awareness, regarding the magnitude of the challenge of mental health, compounding this is a lack of reliable information, with regard to the prevalence of disorders within the communities [21]. Whilst we are seeing ever increasing numbers of Africans seeking out formal mental health services [22].

5. South African context

South Africa remains one of the world's most unequal countries, with areas in which people living still remaining racially divided, even after 25 years of democracy [23]. The result of this division is that there are two economies which coexist in South Africa, the first being one which is not all together dissimilar from that of the global north and then that which is rife with poverty and limitations of access [24]. It would make sense then that the vast majority of South Africans who belong to this second economy would depend on state healthcare. Not dissimilar to many post-colonial societies South Africa has ageing infrastructure within many of its state owned and subsidised sectors. Some of the challenges faced by this sector are not dissimilar to those seen in other parts of the continent such as inconsistent planning for healthcare infrastructure and inadequate allocation of funds [25].

6. Provision of mental health within the South African context

On the continent health is generally poorly funded, and in comparison, to other areas of health, mental health is often more poorly developed [21]. Within Sub-Saharan Africa, mental health services are generally limited to hospital-based services, within the major urban areas. However, within these settings human resources are often limited, with a large population depending on access to these services [20].

It is currently estimated that within the South African context approximately 5% of the health budget is spent specifically on mental health [26]. The vast majority of this budget is spent on curative interventions as opposed to preventative interventions [27]. As such managing healthcare in a reactive as opposed to proactive approach. When these figures were examined on a provincial level, it was found that only a few of the better functioning provinces were keeping within the National allocation of funds for mental health, with some provinces allocating far below this percentage.

There have been several arguments which have been made that some of these provincial departments of health have been struggling to maintain their basic services let alone their infrastructure [28–30]. In some instances, to support these views, it has been highlighted that staff have been failed, in terms of not having received the basic equipment required so as to do their jobs and to conduct their work safely. An example highlighted by [31] was that in Port Elizabeth, one of the largest cities in the Eastern Cape, there is only one state ambulance currently in operation. As highlighted challenges exist with the provision of basic services, which are essential to save lives. As a result, it could be assumed that more specialised and less acute healthcare services could prove to be more difficult.

Again, this is the life experience of the second economy, which is wildly different from that of the former economy. In which we see better patient to staff ratios, newer and well-maintained infrastructure and staff being more appropriately equipped, with required equipment and safety equipment. For this reason, it is important to understand the manner in which people make sense of and experience their worlds.

7. Family therapy within the South African context

In South Africa to become a Psychologist, one has to complete an undergraduate degree, an Honours Program and a Master's degree, after which it is required for you to complete a year internship, board exams and potentially a community service year, depending upon which stream you enter [32]. South Africa currently has five categories in which one can register as a psychologist with the Health Professions Council of South Africa (HPCSA).

Given the duration of time and the associated direct and indirect costs of training, it can already be assumed that the those coming from more resourced backgrounds would be more likely to become psychologists, within the field. Whilst in contrast, the majority of those whom they will attempt to provide services to, even if only in their community service and internships, will be from the aforementioned second economy, which is far less resourced. This experience has been expressed by some authors, that the life of privilege which they have lived had left them feeling isolated from and experienced difficulty in connecting to disadvantaged communities [33].

It has been argued that the development of psychological services for non-white populations was severely stunted by some real and some imagined obstacles [34]. Like the vast majority of psychotherapeutic modalities, family therapy was developed within the Western World and was subsequently imported to the African context [35]. One of the dangers argued in so doing, is the inappropriate application of this model. This potential for inappropriate application is based on imposition of universalism [36]. This universality is grounded in the belief that only one humanity is in existence, and thus there is only one psychology, one philosophy and as such only one way of being [34]. For Morkel [33], she felt that her training had also failed in preparing her to bridge that gap, between her formalised Western training and the needs of the community which she would service.

Whilst the inability to speak client's first languages and to have an intimate first-hand knowledge of their customs and beliefs would be challenging, it can be argued that these would not stop the therapist from being able to provide a level of assistance and or intervention in the here and now [34]. To counter act this, it was suggested that therapist attempt to bring "pscyhotheraputic contexts" to the clients, by attempting to see the world through their lens as opposed to that of a Western one [37]. There has been an argument that South Africa, as a result of its diversity requires a deviation from traditional systemic interventions.

Perhaps this is the most important and valuable stance to have. So as to avoid falling into traps of our own preconceived biases, regarding race and culture, which undoubtedly were influenced by our current and historical context, which we live in currently and grew up in. This is because in apartheid South Africa we were taught to believe that culture is pure, static and unwavering [34]. The result of which was to reproduce and reinforce ethnicity and perpetuate a false ideology of cultural determinism [38]. This as the cultural boundaries which were more clearly defined along racial lines are less clearly defined, in this multicultural society [39, 40].

Considering the mental health and family health needs of the continent, it is believed that family therapy and by extension of this family therapists would be well-suited to intervene, treat and assist [35]. However, as already highlighted there are some real and perceived impediments to the application thereof.

The provision of psychological services and specifically that of family therapy, is limited within the African context [41]. This underdevelopment of these services, are thought to often be similar to other aspects of underdevelopment found in these African countries [22]. However, with the limited number of trained professionals available, this number decreases when we examine the number of therapists who are adequately trained to adapt these skills to the contextual needs of the populations which we service [42]. Whilst we are seeing ever increasing numbers of Africans seeking out formal mental health services, these challenges will need to be addressed in order for these needs to be met [22].

At present there is no registration category of Family Therapist [35]. For this reason, the vast majority of professional practicing family therapy will be psychologists and social workers, who have all undergone various levels of training on the topic. It should also be noted that family therapy is a relatively young field, within the context of Africa, with interest only becoming prevalent in the 60s and 70s in South Africa [35]. This challenge is not unique to South Africa and is rather a challenge seen throughout the continent with no registration category for family or couples' therapists being present throughout the continent, the result of this, is a contribution to the lack of cohesion amongst family therapist on the continent [35].

The question can then be posed, as to whether or not the inefficiency of therapy can be attributed to the family, which is failing to respond, or to the therapist, who is failing to adapt to the family [43]. This could potentially be as a result of the greater focus on the consistency, of application of learned theories, as opposed to the ability to adapt, to the needs to our clients [44].

Family therapy has been noted to have been growing around the world, with Africa being no exception to the global trend [35]. Family therapy places its focus on how to liberate and empower clients [45]. It has been argued that it's collectivist orientation, results in it being considered as contextually appealing to the continent considering the shared cultural collective orientation.

Some models have been adapted to be used within and adapted to the South African context. For example, Seedat and Nell [46] argued that the most appropriate model of family therapy available was that of Jay Hayley's problem-solving therapy [47]. They argued for a six-step intervention, which they believed would be easy to teach, readily accepted by families and practical in its application. These steps would be: Greeting; Socialising; Problem Identification; Bringing the problem into the room; Goal Setting and Contracting, all to be conducted in a session of one hour. It was believed that this would result in the psychologist being able to explore social, psychological and somatoform complaints with the family. The result is a model which lends itself effectively the biopsychosocial model, in which a therapeutic context is generated which holds practical value for both the family and the therapist. Problems become mutual, with the family's views and experiences becoming resources, and being of value. There is also a level of empowerment which occurs, as the family are ultimately developing their own solutions to problems.

Whilst in contrast there have been models which have been developed within the South African context. One such example of this is the Interactional Pattern Analysis (IPA). The underlying assumption is that the quality of our mental health is causally related to the quality of our interpersonal relationships [16]. Emphasis is placed on that which can be observed in the interaction between the individual and their environment [48]. As such an inter-psychic stance is adopted, in which the observable interaction between individual's is the focal point [16]. Bateson [49] argued that interpersonal interactions were based on a trial-and-error system, in which a feedback loop would result [49], with behaviour being modified as a result, leading to self-correction within the system. As a result of this it was argued that individuals would have preferred or more frequently engaged with interactional styles, which could be observed during their interactions with others [50]. As a result of this, the tool of the IPA (Interactional Pattern Analysis) has been designed to guide the psychotherapeutic process whilst also identifying nodal points of the client or patient's interactional style [51] which need to be engaged with so as to result in change from the perturbing of them [52]. It is postulated that this should take place that there will be observable changes in the client or patient's observable behaviour and that there will be a subjective experience of relief for the presenting complaint [48]. This as it is argued that the presentation of symptomatic behaviour, is conceptualised as an adaptive function, within a relational context, which serves the function of maintaining the system [53]. Thus, within this approach the symptomatic behaviour is seen as a function of the individuals' relationship or relationships.

This psycho-diagnostic tool examines sixteen interpersonal variables, from which a description of the observable behaviour will be established, which will allow for the sketching of an individual's interpersonal style [51]. The intervention would then be the link between the clients' patterns of behaviour and their presenting complaints. Based on this connection, relevant and appropriate psychotherapeutic interventions can be implemented [17].

This tool has spawned research focusing on the evaluation and contrasting of the effects of incubator care and kangaroo mother care [54]. It also saw the extensions of it into the realm of child psychotherapy, with the development of Teddy Bear Therapy [55]. This approach has been highlighted to have been effective and of benefit to children who have experienced traumatic events, which can be thought to occur relatively frequently within the South African context [56].

It has also been used to conceptualise and treat Functional Neurological Symptom Disorder (Conversion Disorder), from a systemic and interactional approach [53]. This could be considered putting into clinical practice that which Du Plooy [48] postulated with regards it being used to conceptualise and treat psychologically, mental health conditions.

It has also been used in a preliminary study to assess the incapability of separated couples [57]. Whilst inversely it was also used to assess the subjective levels of marital satisfaction, in a correlational study [58]. It has also been used to assess the effectiveness of therapeutic intervention in preventing the breakdown of partner relationships [59].

8. Conclusion

Family therapy from an African perspective is in a developmental phase, and for this reason limited attention has been paid to families within this context [22]. However, with that having been said African authors are frequently involved in collaborative studies and projects with international academics and clinicians [35]. As highlighted within this chapter there are developments within the field, in Africa. Whilst perhaps these have not been as well published as work originating from the global north, this should also serve as a reminder that whilst implementing and conducting the work that we do, the important role that publication has to allow for this to better known and more accessible.

There is continued need to integrate culture-specific theories and interventions into contemporary Western approaches, so as to meet the needs for this context [22]. However, this appears to be being addressed, as the modality gains popularity within the continent. Though to expedite this process, there is need for improvement with regulation and awareness of the modality [35]. One potential manner in which these objectives could be achieved is through the revival of organisations which promote and support the training in, research in and the supervision within this modality. Whilst the value of specific registration category cannot be discounted, however this is perhaps a longer-term goal, to be addressed at a later stage.

Author details

Barry Lachlan Kevin Viljoen
Department of Psychiatry, Division of Clinical Psychology, The University of the Witwatersrand, Johannesburg, South Africa

*Address all correspondence to: viljoen.barry7@gmail.com

References

[1] Nobles WW. From black psychology to Sakhu Djaer: Implications for the further development of a pan African black psychology. Journal of Black Psychology. 2015;**41**(5):399-414. DOI: 10.1177/0095798415598038

[2] Ratele K. The World Look Like This from Here: Thoughts on African Psychology. Johannesburg, South Africa: Wits University Press; 2019. pp. 1-248

[3] Schwartz R. No Bad Parts. Boulder, Colorado, United States of America: Sounds True; 2021

[4] Metz T, Gaie JBR. The African ethic of Ubuntu/Botho: Implications for research on morality. Journal of Moral Education. 2010;**39**(3):273-290. DOI: 10.1080/03057240.2010.497609

[5] Lutz DW. African Ubuntu philosophy and global management. Journal of Business Ethics. 2009;**84**(3 SUPPL):313-328. DOI: 10.1007/s10551-009-0204-z

[6] Viljoen BLK. Can "Ubuntu" be Used as a Psychotherapeutic Epistemology? Pretoria, South Africa: University of Limpopo; 2015

[7] Nwoye A. What is African psychology the psychology of? Theory & Psychology. 2015b;**25**(1):96-116. DOI: 10.1177/0959354314565116

[8] Nwoye A. African psychology and the Africentric paradigm to clinical diagnosis and treatment. South African Journal of Psychology. 2015a;**45**(3):305-317. DOI: 10.1177/0081246315570960

[9] Mnyaka M, Motlhabi M. The African concept of Ubuntu/Botho and its socio-moral significance. Black Theology. 2005;**3**(2):215-237. DOI: 10.1558/blth.3.2.215.65725

[10] Sodi T, Bopape D, Makgahlela M. Botho as an essential ingredient of African psychology: An insider perspective. South Africa Journal of Psychology. 2021;**2021**:1-12. DOI: 10.1177/0081246320985259

[11] Mangena F. African ethics through Ubuntu: A postmodern exposition. Journal of Pan African Studies. 2016;**9**(2):66-81

[12] Jack-Ide IO, Uys L. Barriers to mental health services utilization in the Niger delta region of Nigeria: Service users' perspectives. Pan African Medical Journal. 2013;**14**:159. DOI: 10.11604/pamj.2013.14.159.1970

[13] Shai M, Sodi T. Pathways to mental health care by members of a rural community in South Africa. 2015. DOI: 10.1080/14330237.2, 13015.1065052

[14] Turner V. Social dramas and stories about them. Critical Inquiry. 1980;**7**(1):141-168

[15] Baumann S. Madness: Stories of Uncertainty and Hope. Cape Town: Jonathan Ball Publishers; 2020. pp. 1-352

[16] Vorster C. General Systems Theory and Psychotherapy: Beyond Post-Modernism. Satori Publishers; 2003

[17] Vorster C. Impact: The Story of Interactional Therapy. Pretoria, South Africa: Satori Publishers; 2011. pp. 1-129

[18] Ware NC, Idoko J, Kaaya S, Biraro IA, Wyatt MA, Agbaji O, et al. Explaining adherence success in sub-Saharan Africa: An ethnographic study. PLoS Medicine. 2009;**6**(1):0039-0047. DOI: 10.1371/journal.pmed.1000011

[19] Saxena S, Thornicroft G, Knapp M, Whiteford H. Resources for mental health: Scarcity, inequity, and inefficiency. Lancet. 2007;**370**(9590):878-889. DOI: 10.1016/S0140-6736(07)61239-2

[20] Ventevogel P, Jordans M, Reis R, De Jong J. Madness or sadness? Local concepts of mental illness in four conflict-affected African communities. Conflict and Health. 2013;**7**(1):1-16. DOI: 10.1186/1752-1505-7-3

[21] Okasha A. Mental health in Africa: The role of the WPA. World Psychiatry. 2002;**1**(1):32-35

[22] Jithoo V, Bakker T. Family therapy within the African context. In: Counseling People of African Ancestry. New York, New York, United States of America: Cambridge University Press; 2011. pp. 142-154. DOI: 10.1017/CBO9780511977350.012

[23] Koka M. Covid-19 exposes inequalities between blacks and whites, experts say. Times Live. 2020. Available from: https://www.timeslive.co.za/news/south-africa/2020-05-10-covid-19-exposes-inequalities-between-blacks-and-whites-experts-say/

[24] Laher S. Editorial : Psychological Assessment in Africa : The Time Is Now ! 1-3. 2019

[25] Human Rights Watch. Africa: Covid-19 Exposes Healthcare Shortfalls. Human Rights Watch: Africa; 2020. Available from: https://www.hrw.org/news/2020/06/08/africa-covid-19-exposes-healthcare-shortfalls

[26] Docrat S, Besada D, Cleary S, Daviaud E, Lund C. Mental health system costs, resources and constraints in South Africa: A national survey. Health Policy and Planning. 2019;**34**(9):706-719. DOI: 10.1093/heapol/czz085

[27] Petersen I, Lund C. Mental health service delivery in South Africa from 2000 to 2010: One step forward, one step back. South African Medical Journal. 2011;**101**(10):751-757

[28] Gwarube S. DA calls for Eastern Cape Department of Health to be placed under administration. DA. 2020. Available from: https://www.da.org.za/2020/06/da-calls-for-eastern-cape-department-of-health-to-be-placed-under-administration#:~:text=The Eastern Cape does not have a functioning health system.&text=As per the Eastern Cape,to all in the province

[29] Ndenze B. DA wants EC Health Department placed in administration. EWN Eyewitness News. 2020. Available from: https://ewn.co.za/2020/06/15/da-wants-ec-health-dept-placed-in-administration

[30] Ntsaluba G, Fana W. Eastern Cape Health Department Is Failing Health Workers, Says Denosa. Johannesburg, South Africa: City Press; 2020. Available from: https://www.news24.com/citypress/news/eastern-cape-health-department-is-failing-health-workers-says-denosa-20200607

[31] Venter S. Eastern Cape Healthcare Has Collapsed: "Sick Poeple Are Fighting Each Other". Johannesburg, South Africa: City Press; 2020. Available from: https://www.news24.com/citypress/news/eastern-cape-healthcare-has-collapsed-sick-people-are-fighting-each-other-20200628

[32] Professional Board of Psychology. 2020. Retrieved 12 April 2020, from: https://www.hpcsa.co.za/

[33] Morkel E. Therapy with children affected by divorce. In: Paper Presented at the 9th SAAMFT International Conference, Durban, South Africa. May 2004

[34] Seedat M, Nell V. Third world or one world: Mysticism, pragmatism, and pain in family therapy in South Africa. South African Journal of Psychology. 2022;**990**(3):141-149

[35] Asiimwe R, Lesch E, Karume M, Blow AJ. Expanding our international reach: Trends in the development of systemic family therapy training and implementation in Africa. Journal of Marital and Family Therapy. 2021;**47**(4):815-830. DOI: 10.1111/jmft.12514

[36] Hook D. Critical Psychology. Cape Town, South Africa: UCT Press; 2004

[37] Lifschitz S. The story of the case, or finding ways to create psychotherapeutic contexts with black clients. In: Mason J, Rubenstein J, editors. Family Therapy in South Africa Today. Durban, South Africa: Congella; 1989

[38] Rohner RP. Toward a conception of culture for cross-cultural psychology. Journal of Cross-Cultural Psychology. 1984;**15**(2):11-138

[39] Jamal A, Kizgin H, Rana NP, Laroche M, Dwivedi YK. Impact of acculturation, online participation and involvement on voting intentions. Government Information Quarterly. **36**(3):510-519. DOI: 10.1016/j.giq.2019.04.001. ISSN 0740-624X

[40] Jolly RJ. Cultured Violence: Narrative, Social Suffering, and Engendering Human Rights in Contemporary South Africa. Vol. 7. Liverpool University Press; 2010. pp. 1-192

[41] Nwoye A, Nwoye CMA. Memory and narrative healing processes in grief work in Africa: Reflections on promotion of re-anchoring. Journal of Family Psychotherapy. 2012;**23**(2):138-158. DOI: 10.1080/08975353.2012.679904

[42] Nwoye A. The shattered microcosm: imperatives for improved family therapy in Africa in the 21st century. 2022

[43] Nelson T, Winawer H, editors. Critical Topics in Family Therapy. New York, New York, United Sates of America: Springer International Publishing; 2014. DOI: 10.1007/978-3-319-03248-1

[44] McNamee S. Promiscuity in the practice of family therapy. Journal of Family Therapy. 2004;**26**:224-244. DOI: 10.1111/j.1467-6427.2004.00280.x

[45] Nwoye A. Family therapy and the pedagogy of the oppressed: Therapeutic use of songs in apartheid South Africa. Australian and New Zealand Journal of Family Therapy. 2018;**39**(2):200-217. DOI: 10.1002/anzf.1297

[46] Seedat M, Nell V. Third world or one world: Mysticism, pragmatism, and pain in family therapy in South Africa. South African Journal of Psychology. 1990;**20**(3):141-149. DOI: 10.1177/008124639002000302

[47] Haley J. Problem-Solving Therapy. San Francisco, California, United States of America: Jossey-Bass Publishers; 1976. pp. 1-288

[48] du Plooy K. Interactional therapy : Prospects for treating mental health conditions. Journal of Psychology in South Africa. 2019;**0237**(29):630-637. DOI: 10.1080/14330237.2019.1689461

[49] Bateson G. Mind and Nature: A Necessary Unit. New York, New York, United Sates of America: Fontana; 1979

[50] Jackson D. The individual and the larger context. Family Process. 1967;**6**(2):139-147

[51] Vorster C, Roos V, Beukes M. A psycho-diagnostic tool for

psychotherapy: Interactional pattern analysis (IPA). Journal of Psychology in Africa. 2014;**23**(3):525-530

[52] du Plooy K. The Use of the Interactional Pattern Analysis as a Tool for Effective Short Term Psychotherapy among Students at South African Tertiary Institutions. Pretoria, South Africa; 2016. Available from: https://www.researchgate.net/publication/307607574

[53] Dennis LAM, Phipps WD. Functional neurological symptom disorder (conversion disorder) from an interactional approach: A composite case study. Australian and New Zealand Journal of Family Therapy. 2020;**41**(4):310-324. DOI: 10.1002/anzf.1434

[54] Green SL, Phipps WD. Interactional pattern analysis of mother – baby pairs: Kangaroo mother care versus incubator care. South African Journal of Psychology. 2015;**45**(2):194-207. DOI: 10.1177/0081246314565961

[55] Beyers L, Phipps WD, Vorster C. An introduction to teddy bear therapy: A systems family therapy approach to child Psychotheraoy. Journal of Family Psychotherapy. 2017;**28**(4):317-332. DOI: 10.1080/08975353.2017.1301156

[56] Baloyi L. Teddy bear therapy : An application : Research article. Child Abuse Research in South Africa. 2006;**7**(2):17-25

[57] Hughes J. A Preliminary Study to Assess the Incompatibility of Separated South African Couples Using the Interactional Pattern Analysis. Pretoria, South Africa: University of Limpopo; 2014

[58] Kasseepursad A. Interactional Pattern Analyses and Subjective Levels of Marital Satisfaction: A Correlational Study. Pretoria, South Africa: University of Limpopo; 2011

[59] Nell E. The Effect of a DVD Counselling Programme in Preventing the Breakdown of Partner Relationships of Master's Students in Clinical Psychology. Pretoria, South Africa: University of Limpopo; 2010

Chapter 4

Perspective Chapter: Helping BIPOC LGBTQIA+ Families through Inclusive Therapy and Advocacy

Lucy Parker-Barnes, Noel McKillip and Carolyn Powell

Abstract

Families are phenomenological and unique. All families are valuable, but historically, many family types have been underrepresented. Families with members who identify in the BIPOC LGBTQIA+ communities have historically been underrepresented and marginalized. Helping BIPOC LGBTQIA+ families involves both clinical work and advocacy. Advocacy for the professional identity of counseling, marriage and family therapy, and related helpers involves various aspects. These aspects include leadership theory and integration, importance of professional identity, the need to continue to infuse multiculturalism within the counseling and family therapy identities, and continued skills for counselors to learn inclusive advocacy. Skills and implications for advocacy as they relate to clients who intersect among the LGBTQAI+ and BIPOC communities, will be described.

Keywords: family counseling, inclusive counseling, multiculturalism, BIPOC, LGBTQIA+, BIPOC LGBTQIA+ families

1. Introduction

Advocacy and leadership have become increasingly recognized, in part, due to the growth of knowledge and awareness from leaders in the family counseling fields [1]. Leadership theories and types have evolved from a traditionally innate sense of personality to a now more explicitly learned set of competences that counselors and family therapists use with increased intentionality. Leadership, specifically, is now seen by helpers as not a single action, but rather an on-going dialog or a learned set of skills or behaviors [1–3]. Counselors and family therapists must focus on increasing their professional leadership, identity, and advocacy to best help all family types.

Definitions of leadership in family counseling have expanded to include cultural responsivity and social justice [4, 5]. Cultural responsivity includes cultural sensitivity, cultural knowledge, cultural empathy, cultural guidance, and, most recently, cultural humility [6, 7]. Similarly, social justice is increasingly being incorporated into counselor education, counseling psychology, and marriage and family counseling literature [8]. To date, however, there is still limited understanding, research, and enactment of social justice measures in all these related fields [9]. Of the knowledge currently enacted, scholars have identified multiple sub-constructs of social justice, including affirmative action, emphasis on equality, decolonization, and disruption of marginalization, oppression, and inequality [9]. In the below documentation, various aspects of leadership skills and ideas will be described as they relate to multiculturalism and inclusive advocacy. These types could also be applied to underrepresented clients and families, including BIPOC LGBTQIA+ families.

2. Traditional leadership theories in family counseling

Various leadership theories drive different forms of advocacy in family counseling. Leadership theories efficacious for family therapists and counselors include: 1) Trait Theories, 2) Behavior Theories, 3) Contingency Theories, 4) Path-Goal Theory, 5) Leader-Membership Exchange Theory, and 6) Supervision Leadership models [10, 11]. Though each of these leadership theories is different, each theory can be effective depending on congruency to a counselor's, family therapist's, or leader's personality and preferred leadership style. For example, Trait Leadership Theory includes various salient traits of a family counselor leader, such as extraversion and emotional intelligence. Comparatively, other Behavioral Theories focus on behaviors learned and used by effective leaders, rather than on personality or emotion-based traits, alone. Additionally, Contingency Theories focus on traits and behaviors, as well as context and other significant relational factors (e.g., sociocultural considerations) with those whom family counselors will serve and lead [10]. Additionally considered is Supervision Leadership, which uses culturally responsive leadership models and practices [11]. One of the greatest improvements in family counseling and other counseling fields includes the increase of educating colleagues and trainees about the need to incorporate all leadership models with culturally responsive and just components. Recently, leaders in the field have begun incorporating the Socially Just and Culturally Responsive Counseling Leadership Model (SJCRCLM) in addition to the recently described models [11]. This chapter will emphasize ideas congruent with the SJCRCLM designed for clients and families in the BIPOC LGBTQIA+ community.

3. Importance of inclusive leadership practices

To supplement professional identity and leadership modeling, leaders in family counseling and related fields must also understand and establish ethical and culturally relevant practices in those fields [12]. The American Association for Marriage and Family Therapy (AAMFT) Code of Ethics emphasizes inclusiveness and diversity in many ways, including diversity being listed as one of AAMFT's main aspirational core values [13]. Furthermore, the International Association of Marriage and Family Counselors (IAMFC) and American Counseling Association (ACA) also explicitly mention valuing diversity and cultural competency [12]. Furthermore, the ACA's Code of Ethics requires that counselors be continuously ethically and culturally competent. These competencies are specifically aligned in Standards A.2.c., B.1.a, C.2.f, E.5.b., E.8., F.2.b., F. 11.c. and H.5.d [12]. Culturally relevant history that need to be increasingly taught in family counseling programs include the development of the Association of Non-White Concerns (ANWC) in 1985, the development of the Multicultural

Counseling Competencies and Standards (MCCS) published in 1992, the formation of the Association for Lesbian, Gay, Bisexual, and Transgender Issues in Counseling (i.e., SAIGE, then known as AGLBIC) in 1997, and others [10]. Family counselors must also recall the ACA Code of Ethics: Standard E.5.c, which is to "recognize historical and social prejudices...." While critical social justice efforts are gaining awareness, multiculturally competent advocacy for clients and professionals remain lacking. Thus, ultimately, family therapists and counselors must all embrace their organization's professional identity, which each include to best serve clients of all cultures. As mentioned, infusing the SJCRCLM and adapting traditional leadership and service models to be increasingly inclusive is a need in all related mental health fields.

4. Assessing family counselor culturally relevant leadership practices

Both trainees as well as seasoned professionals should be encouraged to consistently create an affirming clinical environment by teaching about the effects of context, semantics, and positions of privilege [14]. Usage of assessments and group dialog in family work can be increasingly helpful to understand some of these systemic factors [15]. One such assessment that can be used in family counseling or individual counseling supervision is the Multicultural Competencies Self-Assessment Survey or related multicultural surveys [16]. Another professional advocacy assessment includes the Advocacy Competencies Self-Assessment Survey, which helps counseling trainees or counselors assess their capabilities of being advocates and culturally focused versus lacking in these areas [17]. Administration of the above assessments are two potential ways to address both client and professional advocacy using a systemic and cultural emphasis. Another culturally relevant and ethical practice needed by family counselors is the continued establishment and maintenance of ethical boundaries (ACA, 2014; CACREP, 2016). Specifically, per the 2014 ACA Code of Ethics, family and individual counselors are required to establish and maintain differentiated boundaries between their personal and professional roles, especially when implicit biases due to cultural differences may exist [12, 18]. In all family sessions, boundaries of the family counselor need to be distinguished, rather than left tacit and confusing. Sometimes, due to the systemic nature of families, dual roles may occur; however, all roles should be navigated with caution, consultation, and clear communication. Other culturally inclusive ethical strategies include modeling being an advocate for multicultural awareness, facilitating in-session activities about family and culture, and emphasizing the need for cultural awareness in supervision, class, and clinical practice [10, 19].

5. Advocacy to address salient socio-political issues affecting LGBTQIA+ clients and families

Client advocacy is another needed leadership skill for family counselors [10]. It is imperative that clinicians remember the term "multicultural" is inclusive of issues relating beyond outward differences alone [20]. With understanding that identity transcends beyond phenotype, family counselors must be advocates for all individuals of a family, especially those who are marginalized in larger society. For example, due to recent legislative policies, one demographic of people who are still marginalized in current society includes people identifying as, Gay, Bisexual, Transgender, Queer/ Questioning, Intersex, or Asexual (LGBTQIA+) [10, 20]. With same-sex marriage recently legalized in the United States, individuals often forget that discrimination toward LGBTQIA+ people has not ceased in America. One example that exemplifies how individuals in the LGBTQIA+ group are still unjustly marginalized, is the example of recent formation of discriminatory legislation, Florida House Bill 1557 or otherwise known as the "Don't Say Gay Bill." This Bill states that classroom instruction about sexual orientation or gender identity may not occur at all in Kindergarten through Grade Three [21]. Additionally, as of 2022, at least three states in America, including Georgia, Florida, and Alabama do not ban conversion therapy [22]. Not long ago, too, in 2016, former Governor, Bill Haslam of Tennessee, signed a law into place that allowed private practice family or individual counselors to not have to work with clients of whom they disagree with ideologically, religiously, or regarding sexual orientation, despite the client's presenting issues or need [23, 24]. More specifically, counselors in Tennessee, who may be approached with clients who are gay and with a presenting issue, such as severe depression or suicidality, may refer out this counseling seeking client, only due to disagreeing with his, her, hir, or their lifestyle, sexuality and/or gender expression, alone [23, 24]. This Bill is denounced The American Counseling Association. However, despite professional advocacy, this Bill symbolizes the large margin of current advocacy work that is still needed in the counseling profession. Thus, in many areas of the United States, clients in the BIPOC and LGTBQIA+ population are still marginalized.

6. Intersection of BIPOC and LGBTQIA+

LGBTQIA+ individuals who are also racial/ethnic minorities are multi-marginalized and are often subject to microaggressions associated with the intersection of their two historically oppressed identities [25]. On average, sexual minority people of color experience less support, greater stress, and fewer resources than White LGBTQIA+ individuals [26]. BIPOC LGBTQIA+ members also experience increased family rejection [27] and have a greater tendency to conceal their sexual orientation [28]. These "double minority" individuals encounter mental health challenges linked to sexism, racism, cis-heteronormativity, and challenges related to oppression toward their intersecting identities. While culture and community connections (including the presence of role models and family/peer support) improve resiliency, fears of "losing face," unwillingness to disclose ill health, and mental health providers' lack of cultural competency, create barriers to effective mental health support for these individuals with these intersecting identities [10]. Considering the disparity of services provided to BIPOC LGBTQIA+ identifying individuals and their families, it is crucial that family counselors advocate. Additionally, family counselors need to continue to learn to adequately conceptualize the unique variation of overlapping identities when beginning work with any new client of family. Relatedly, sexual, and racial minorities make up a disproportionately large percentage of the United States' incarcerated population. Black males make up approximately 13 percent of the population, yet account for 34 percent of the total male prison population [29]. In 2017, 9.3 percent of men and 35.7 percent of women in prison identified as sexual minorities, compared to less than 4 percent of incarcerated White women within the U.S. Additionally, gay Black men have twice the incarceration rate compared to their White, non-racial minority counterparts [29]. Since individuals who face the dual minority status of being both a racial and sexual minority face a significantly disproportionate risk of jail time, it is critical that family counselors recognize the disparity and advocate with these clients. Risk of incarceration is only one marginalization experienced for clients and families identifying within the BIPOC and LGBTQIA+ community. A growing body of evidence documents the negative effects of racism on the emotional, psychological, and physiological functioning of BIPOC families [30]. Psychological distress (e.g., anxiety, depressive symptoms) due to perceived racial discrimination is more prevalent among BIPOC students and families than their White peers and families [31]. Other barriers include, racial injustice, and discriminatory practices in schools, workplaces and [32, 33]. Additionally, Black mothers have higher rates of preterm births, indicating higher risks for health complications among Black children from the start of life [34]. Once born, Black children are also less frequently exposed to culturally appropriate childcare and are often racially profiled as aggressive in various arenas, which often escalates into more police-based discrimination as these children age [35–37]. Considering all these stressors and traumas, BIPOC families frequently endure ambiguous, non-death losses, or "losses that remain unclear and thus without resolution," such as historical trauma, below-average academic opportunities, and oppressive laws and policies [38]. Thus, effective professional family counselors must learn to employ a trauma-informed and culturally responsive modality for BIPOC LGBTQIA+ clients and their families.

7. Leadership and family counseling strategies as advocacy

Advocating for BIPOC LGBTQIA+ individuals and their families by refuting punitive and discriminatory legislation such as Florida Bill 1557 and Tennessee Bill 1556, as well as intervening and preventing less covert and overt acts, is needed by all family counselors. Speaking with legislators and other public individuals is a crucial advocacy component that is needed by clinicians in our field, but not currently mandated. These actions are rooted in family counseling education and the AAMFT and ACA Code of Ethics. As counselors and related mental health clinicians have mentioned prior, when counselors see oppression, we must accept responsibility for individual and collective social action. Various systemic related resources for family counselors and their family clients include the following:

1. **Psychoeducation** Family counselors seeking consultation about increased knowledge is needed. Additionally, family counselors who provide psychoeducation to BIPOC LGBTQIA+ families are also needed. For example, prior researchers have found that biracial children often experience more identity-confusion when White parents do not foster their Black identity development [39]. Opposite of minimizing a child's ethnicity, family counselors should encourage parents in these families to reflect their biracial or BIPOC child's ethnic strengths and marginalized identity [40]. One concrete resource that can be used among family counselors is called The Safe Place [41]. The Safe Place is a free app that was created by Jasmin Pierre in 2018. The Safe Place is focused on psychoeducation and self-care for people who identify in the Black community [4, 41]. The Safe Place is geared toward the Black community and initially invites group discussion about mental health. Users of this app can navigate different parts of the application to see features such as, Black mental health prevalence and statistics, ways to cope, ways to engage in self-care, ways to cope after experiencing or witnessing police brutality, suggestions for meditation and ways to seek additional support through nontherapeutic resources such as, church or through

suggestions of mental health professionals. More information about The Safe Place can be found here: https://blackgirlnerds.com/minority-mental-health-app-the-safe-place. Additionally, a recent meditation application called Liberate: Black Meditation App is a free app designed specifically for the BIPOC community and led by BIPOC teachers. Liberate was designed by Julio A Rivera in 2018 to provide wellness support for people from the BIPOC community. This app provides meditations for users, along with videos of hope and insight from yoga instructors and other contributors. Meditations specifically designed to help users deal with microaggressions and trauma related to societal racism are also utilized. Other meditations are also designed to help users embrace, reconnect, and honor their often-underrepresented varying heritages. More information about Liberate can be found here: https://www.washingtonpost.com/lifestyle/magazine/think-meditation-could-help-cope-with-microaggressions-theres-an-app-for-that/2020/03/31/b28ba252-5fb8-11ea-b014-4fafa866bb81_story.html

2. Being Trauma Informed Family counselors need to continue to learn how to help families dealing with trauma related to intersecting isms. Various isms that BIPOC LGBTQIA+ families may experience, include lack of physical access to resources due to discrimination, overt and covert racism, sexism, homophobia, transphobia, and chronic microaggressions [4, 25, 42]. A specific traumatic occurrence that impacts BIPOC LGBTQIA+ communities is police brutality [42]. As of 2020, BIPOC were killed at least 1.6 times the rate of their White peers. Additionally, Black men and Native American men were killed at almost 3 times the rate of White men by police. Family counselors should consider both the psychological and physical wounds that police brutality may trigger for many BIPOC and BIPOC LGBTQIA+ clients and families [42]. Furthermore, typical broadcasting does not usually cover the hate-crimes, violence, and grief related to oppressions surrounding BIPOC LGBTQIA+ communities. Being trauma-informed and having cultural competence, humility, composure, quick wittedness, creativity, persistence, assertiveness, and resilience are all ingredients of successful family counselors [43]. Family counseling that already intentionally incorporates trauma has already proven beneficial in recent literature [44].

3. Recognizing Representation Family counselors need to help mitigate the lack of representation that many BIPOC LGBTQIA+ members and families experience in mental health support and healing services. BIPOC, LGBTQIA+, and BIPOC LGBTQIA+ folks are often excluded from public media, as well as media surrounding grief and loss support [45, 46]. For example, a protective factor and supportive organization for many clients and families includes the Trevor Project. The Trevor Project is the largest suicide and crisis prevention intervention program for LGBTQIA+ youth in the world. Though this organization is very helpful, many clients in the BIPOC LGBTQIA+ community have shared that this organization, too, lacks representation as it was catalyzed primarily by Trevor, a White fictional character [47]. Thus, for family counselors to recognize the loss of Trevor and helpfulness of the Trevor Project, while also recognizing the impact of lack of representation on all BIPOC LGBTQIA+ individuals in this and other organizations, is crucial. Increasing representation not only includes representation of BIPOC LGBTQIA+ families and individuals, but also family counselors as advocates.

4. Advocacy Outside of the Counseling Session Family counselors can act as advocates by talking with legislators about terminating discriminatory Bills such as the: Tennessee Bill 1556 Senate Bill (i.e. which does not require counselors to help families or clients who conflict with their religious beliefs), Missouri Senate Bill 1721 (i.e. which prohibits anyone from gender reassignment surgical procedures under age 18), Georgia Senate Bill 368 (i.e. which excludes LGBTQIA+ foster parents from adopting when placement of a child violates certain religious or moral convictions of the fostering agency), Arkansas Stop CRT Act of 2021 (i.e. which would defund and prohibit efforts to teach about history though non-White lenses, like Critical Race Theory), and HR6243 No More Free Ride Act (i.e. prohibiting Federal public benefits for or naturalization of any person who received a payment pursuant or related sources) and others [4, 21, 22]. Family counselors are encouraged to pursue a congruence between their prosocial behaviors in both their professional and personal selves.

5. Increasing Competence and Providing Supportive Resources to Families Family counselors are also expected to help families find physical and psychological support in and outside of the counseling session. Organizations in support of BIPOC LGBTQIA+ affirming counselors, community families, and community members include, but are not limited to 1) the Society for Sexual, Affectional, Intersex, and Gender Expansive Identities (SAIGE), 2) National Queer and Trans Therapists of Color Network (NQTTCN), 3) The National Black Justice Coalition (NBJC), and 4) The National Center for Transgender Equality (NCTE). SAIGE is a division of the American Counseling Association which offers information and support for both counselors in the LGBTQIA+ community and their allies [48]. Another impactful organization, the NQTTCN is a nonprofit agency formed in 2016 that provides support and therapeutic services to queer and transgender people of color (QTPoC) [4]. Additionally, The National Black Justice Coalition (NBJC) is a federal civil rights-based group that was founded in 2003 and focuses on empowering Black lesbian, gay, bisexual, transgender, queer+, and same gender loving people. The NBJC engages in advocacy for federal policy change, research, and education [4]. Family counselors educating themselves, professionally, through groups, such as the NBJC is encouraged. Additionally, family counselors providing these names of supportive groups to family clients may also provide education, universality, and hope. Another influential entity is the National Center for Transgender Equality (NCTE). The NCTE is a social justice organization founded in 2003 that advocates for transgender and nonbinary people [4]. The NCTE facilitates a variety of developments, including the Racial and Economic Justice Initiative (REJI), which advocates for change for transgender people of color experiencing rural and urban poverty (among other obstacles). These are only four of various emerging advocacy groups where family counselors can collaborate and connect clients and families.

8. Conclusion

As referenced throughout this documentation, family counselors' inclusive and multicultural based advocacy, leadership, and clinical practice are needed when working with underrepresented families, especially BIPOC LGBTQIA+ families. Leadership theories and types have evolved and continue to influence the work that family counselors do in this and other areas. Unfortunately, in theory, there will always be societal constraints and power inequities; because of these inequities, however, there will always be a reason for family counselors to unite professionally and clinically advocate for BIPOC LGBTQIA+ families!

Acknowledgements

The authors would like to thank all Northern Illinois University and Northwestern mentors who encouraged advocacy and passion for this subject!

Conflict of interest

The authors declare no conflict of interest.

Author details

Lucy Parker-Barnes[1*], Noel McKillip[2] and Carolyn Powell[2]

1 Gannon University, United States

2 Northwestern University, United States

*Address all correspondence to: parkerba001@gannon.edu

References

[1] Dollarhide CT, Gibson DM, Moss JM. Professional identity development of counselor education doctoral students. Counselor Education and Supervision. 2013;**52**(2):137-150. DOI: 10.1002/j. 1556-6978.2013.00034.x

[2] Hunnicutt Hollenbaugh KM. Increasing leadership behaviors in counselor education doctoral students via study abroad experiences: A single case study approach. Journal of Counselor Leadership and Advocacy. 2015;**2**(2): 170-183. DOI: 10.1080/2326716X.2015. 1066277

[3] Hays DG, Crockett SA, Michel R. A grounded theory of counselor educators' academic leadership development. Counselor Education and Supervision. 2021;**60**(1):51-72. DOI: 10.1002/ ceas.12196

[4] Parker-Barnes L, McKillip N, Powell C. Systemic advocacy for BIPOC LGBTQIA+ clients and their families. The Family Journal. 2022;**30**(3):479-486. DOI: 10.664807221090947

[5] Peters HC, Luke M, Bernard J, Trepal H. Socially just and culturally responsive leadership within counseling and counseling psychology: A grounded theory investigation. The Counseling Psychologist. 2020;**48**(7):953-985. DOI: 10.1177%2F0011000020937431

[6] Levant RF, Wong YJ, American Psychological Association, editors. The Psychology of Men and Masculinities. Washington, DC: American Psychological Association; 2017

[7] Hook JN, Davis DE, Owen J, Worthington EL Jr, Utsey SO. Cultural humility: Measuring openness to culturally diverse clients. Journal of Counseling Psychology. 2013;**60**(3):353. DOI: 10.1037/a0032595

[8] Morrison T, Ferris Wayne M, Harrison T, Palmgren E, Knudson-Martin C. Learning to embody a social justice perspective in couple and family therapy: A grounded theory analysis of MFTs in training. Contemporary Family Therapy. 2022;**4(1)**:1-4. DOI: 10.1007/ s10591-022-09635-8

[9] Goodman LA, Wilson JM, Helms JE, Greenstein N, Medzhitova J. Becoming an advocate: Processes and outcomes of a relationship-centered advocacy training model. The Counseling Psychologist. 2018;**46**(2):122-153. DOI: 10.1177/00110 00018757168

[10] Chang CY, Minton CA, Dixon AL, Myers JE, Sweeney TJ. Professional counseling excellence through leadership and advocacy. Routledge/Taylor & Francis Group; 2012

[11] Peters HC, Luke M. Supervision of leadership model: An integration and extension of the discrimination model and socially just and culturally responsive counseling leadership model. Journal of Counselor Leadership and Advocacy. 2021;**8**(1):71-86. DOI: 10.1080/2326716X.2021.1875341

[12] Kaplan DM, Francis PC, Hermann MA, Baca JV, Goodnough GE, Hodges S, et al. New concepts in the 2014 ACA code of ethics. Journal of Counseling & Development. 2017;**95**(1):110-120 Available from: https://www.apa.org/ethics/code/

[13] Ryder R, Hepworth J. AAMFT ethical code: "Dual relationships". Journal of Marital and Family Therapy.

1990;**16**(2):127-132. DOI: 10.1111/j.1752-0606.1990.tb00833.x

[14] Hurt-Avila KM, Castillo J. Accreditation, professional identity development, and professional competence: A discriminant analysis. Journal of Counselor Leadership and Advocacy. 2017;**4**(1):39-51. DOI: 10.1080/2326716X.2017.1282331

[15] Bevly C, Loseu S, Prosek EA. Infusing social justice advocacy in supervision coursework. Journal of Counselor Leadership and Advocacy. 2017;**4**(1):28-38. DOI: 10.1080/2326716X.2017.1282330

[16] Jones JM, Lee LH. Multicultural competency building: A multi-year study of trainee self-perceptions of cultural competence. Contemporary School Psychology. 2021;**25**(3):288-298. DOI: 10.1007/s40688-020-00339-0

[17] Bvunzawabaya B. Social justice counseling: establishing psychometric properties for the advocacy competencies self-assessment survey© [Doctoral dissertation]. Available from: http://hdl.handle.net/10415/3369

[18] Brew L, Cervantes JM, Shepard D. Millennial counselors and the ethical use of facebook. Professional Counselor. 2013;**3**(2):93-104. DOI: 10.15241/lbb.3.2.93

[19] Ikiz FE, Asici E. The relationship between individual innovativeness and psychological well-being: The example of Turkish counselor trainees. International Journal of Progressive Education. 2017;**13**(1):52-63 Available from: http://www.inased.org/ijpe.htm

[20] Troutman O, Packer-Williams C. Moving beyond CACREP standards: Training counselors to work competently with LGBT clients. The Journal of Counselor Preparation and Supervision. 2014;**6**(1):3. DOI: 10.7729/51.1088

[21] Young C. Florida's 'Don't Say Gay' Bill Inflames the Culture Wars. Available from: https://policycommons.net/artifacts/2299290/floridas-dont-say-gay-bill-inflames-the-culture-wars/3059817/

[22] Movement Advancement Project. Conversion "therapy" Laws. Available from: https://www.lgbtmap.org/equality-maps/conversion_therapy

[23] Ginicola MM, Smith C, Filmore JM, editors. Developing competence in working with LGBTQI+ communities: Awareness, knowledge, skills, and action. Affirmative Counseling with LGBTQI+ People. Alexandria, Virginia: American Counseling Association; 2017:1-20

[24] Smith LC, Okech JE. Ethical issues raised by CACREP accreditation of programs within institutions that disaffirm or disallow diverse sexual orientations. Journal of Counseling & Development. 2016;**94**(3):252-264. DOI: 10.1002/jcad.12082

[25] Balsam KF, Molina Y, Beadnell B, Simoni J, Walters K. Measuring multiple minority stress: The LGBT people of color microaggressions scale. Cultural Diversity and Ethnic Minority Psychology. 2011;**17**(2):163. DOI: 10.1037/a0023244

[26] Toomey RB, Huynh VW, Jones SK, Lee S, Revels-Macalinao M. Sexual minority youth of color: A content analysis and critical review of the literature. Journal of Gay & Lesbian Mental Health. 2017;**21**(1):3-1. DOI: 10.1080/19359705.2016.1217499

[27] Ryan C, Huebner D, Diaz RM, Sanchez J. Family rejection as a predictor of negative health outcomes in white and

Latino lesbian, gay, and bisexual young adults. Pediatrics. 2009;**123**(1):346-352. DOI: 10.1542/peds.2007-3524

[28] Moradi B, Wiseman MC, DeBlaere C, Goodman MB, Sarkees A, Brewster ME, et al. LGB of color and white individuals' perceptions of heterosexist stigma, internalized homophobia, and outness: Comparisons of levels and links. The Counseling Psychologist. 2010;**38**(3):397-424. DOI: 10.1177/0011000009335263

[29] Wildeman C, Wang EA. Mass incarceration, public health, and widening inequality in the USA. The Lancet. 2017;**389**(10077):1464-1474. DOI: 10.1016/S0140-6736(17)30259-3

[30] Chao RC, Mallinckrodt B, Wei M. Co-occurring presenting problems in African American college clients reporting racial discrimination distress. Professional Psychology: Research and Practice. 2012;**43**(3):199. DOI: 10.1037/a0027861

[31] Robinson-Perez A, Marzell M, Han W. Racial microaggressions and psychological distress among undergraduate college students of color: Implications for social work practice. Clinical Social Work Journal. 2020;**48**(4):343-350. DOI: 10.1007/s10615-019-00711-5

[32] Jones SC, Neblett Jr EW. The impact of racism on the mental health of people of color. In: Williams MT, Rosen D, Kanter J, editors. Eliminating Race-Based Mental Health Disparities. Oakland, CA: New Harbinger Books; 2019:79-98

[33] Jones SC, Anderson RE, Gaskin-Wasson AL, Sawyer BA, Applewhite K, Metzger IW. From "crib to coffin": Navigating coping from racism-related stress throughout the lifespan of Black Americans. American Journal of Orthopsychiatry. 2020;**90**(2):267. DOI: 10.1037/ort0000430

[34] Mehra R, Boyd LM, Magriples U, Kershaw TS, Ickovics JR, Keene DE. Black pregnant women "Get the Most Judgment": A qualitative study of the experiences of Black women at the intersection of race, gender, and pregnancy. Women's Health Issues. 2020;**30**(6):484-492. DOI: 10.1016/j.whi.2020.08.001

[35] Gee GC, Walsemann KM, Brondolo E. A life course perspective on how racism may be related to health inequities. American Journal of Public Health. 2012;**102**(5):967-974. DOI: 10.2105/AJPH.2012.300666

[36] James C, Iruka I. Delivering on the Promise of Effective Early Childhood Education. Washington, DC: National Black Child Development Institute; 2018

[37] Stewart EA, Baumer EP, Brunson RK, Simons RL. Neighborhood racial context and perceptions of police-based racial discrimination among black youth. Criminology. 2009;**47**(3):847-887. DOI: 10.1111/j.1745-9125.2009.00159.x

[38] Harris DL, editor. Non-death loss and grief: Context and clinical implications. Routledge. 2019;**1**(1):370-371. ISBN: 9781138320826

[39] Robinson-Wood T, Muse C, Hewett R, Balogun-Mwangi O, Elrahman J, Nordling A, et al. Regular white people things: The presence of white fragility in interracial families. Family Relations. 2021;**70**(4):973-992. DOI: 10.1111/fare.12549

[40] Arredondo P, Avilés RM, Zalaquett CP, Grazioso MD, Bordes V, Hita L, et al. The psychohistorical approach in family counseling with Mestizo/Latino immigrants: A continuum and synergy of worldviews. The Family Journal. 2006;**14**(1):13-27. DOI: 10.1177/1066480705283089

[41] LaSure-Bryant D. Counseling BIPOC students in higher education: Practicing beyond COVID [Virtual Conference: PowerPoint]. Maryland Social Justice Counseling Association, Virtual Conference; 2021. Available from: https://mdcounselorsmcsj.wixsite.com/mcsj

[42] Graham A, Haner M, Sloan MM, Cullen FT, Kulig TC, Jonson CL. Race and worrying about police brutality: The hidden injuries of minority status in America. Victims & Offenders. 2020;**15**(5):549-573. DOI: 10.1080/15564886.2020.1767252

[43] James RK, Gilliland BE. Crisis Intervention Strategies. Cengage Learning. Belmont, CA: Brooks and Cole; 2016

[44] Moir MB. Addressing the Development of Selves in LGBTQIA+ Individuals: A Voice Dialogue Perspective. Pacifica Graduate Institute. 2018;**1**(1):45-47. Available from: https://www.proquest.com/openview/f1042903861125a074fdc067421877b8/1?pq-origsite=gscholar&cbl=18750

[45] Gregory G. Queering suicide: Complicated discourses, compiled deviances, and communal directives surrounding LGBTQIA+ intentional self-initiated death. The Interne. 2019;**1**(1):21-28. Available from: https://scholar.colorado.edu/concern/undergraduate_honors_theses/gm80hv700

[46] Ahmed S. Affective economies. Social Text. 2004;**22**(2):117-139 Available from: https://muse.jhu.edu/article/55780

[47] Green AE, Price-Feeney M, Dorison SH, Pick CJ. Self-reported conversion efforts and suicidality among US LGBTQ youths and young adults, 2018. American Journal of Public Health. 2020;**110**(8):1221-1227. DOI: 10.2105/AJPH.2020.305701

[48] Rose JS, DuFresne RM. Introduction to the special issue advocacy and social justice for LGBTGEQIAP+. Journal of LGBT Issues in Counseling. 2020;**14**(4):290-292. DOI: 10.1080/15538605.2020.1830644

Chapter 5

Intergenerational Attachment Styles, Emotional Regulation and Relational Outcomes in Couples Therapy

Maliha Ibrahim, Manjushree Palit and Rhea Matthews

Abstract

This chapter focuses on the theoretical basis behind intergenerational attachment styles and how they present in romantic relationships. In this chapter, we review the conceptual literature on attachment styles, their development and maintenance across the lifespan. We also explore the role of mutual emotional regulation in disrupting relational distress and improving relationship functioning. We proceed to synthesise efficacy studies and evidence-based research on relational interventions with couples, most commonly presenting concerns in couples therapy and the role of couples therapy in improving romantic relationships across cultural contexts, gender and sexuality identifications. We summarise what has worked, with whom and why while reviewing the various measures and types of clinical interventions offered to couples and report on change scores in outcomes of attachment avoidance/anxiety, relational conflict, relationship functioning and partner satisfaction. Finally, the book chapter presents three case studies with South-Asian couples across diverse life stages, relationship statuses, gender identities and sexual orientations using attachment-based and emotion-focused interventions.

Keywords: attachment, intergenerational, relationships, emotion-focused therapy, Gottman method

1. Introduction

Attachment theory is based on the premise that an infant and caregiver form a bonded relationship. John Bowlby proposed that an infant's innate behavioural tendencies are driven by a biologically-based, motivational system called attachment [2]. The organisation of the attachment behavioural systems involves the following three components–behavioural, emotional, and cognitive [2–4]. An infant separated from a caregiver, experiences intense distress and goes to extraordinary lengths-cries, clings and searches for the attachment figure to prevent separation and re-establish proximity. Therefore, the infant's goal-oriented behavioural tendencies such as seeking proximity with the caregiver are a biologically-driven, motivational system. The intense distress represents the activation of the emotional component of attachment. Separation from a caregiver leads to an intense state of arousal and anxiety, whereas proximity evokes positive emotions. Emotions provide self-regulatory functions in the attachment behavioural system [5]. Finally, attachment behavioural systems include the cognitive component, such as, the infant's mental representation of the attachment figure, self, and the environment [3, 4]. Ainsworth proposed that the infant also uses the attachment figure as a secure base from which to explore the environment, a critical component of attachment. During the first year of the infant's life, the infant learns to maintain the delicate balance between attachment and exploration through assessment of the environment and availability of the attachment figure. In times of distress, the attachment behavioural systems are activated and exploration ceases, whereas when the infant is confident of the availability of the attachment figure, playful exploration of the environment increases [6]. Overall, the activation of the attachment behavioural system is evolutionarily designed to enhance the infant's survival [3, 4].

Research questions

- What is the nature of the relationship between attachment in early years, the formation of attachment styles, and its impact on romantic relationships with partners?
- What is the role played by an individual's emotional regulation and capacity for mutual regulation with one's partner?
- What are some of the key evidence-based psychotherapy models that utilise intergenerational attachment and relational techniques in assessment and intervention with couples?
- What is the efficacy for these models- what works, with whom, in what contexts, and why?
- What is the scope for these evidence-based models with South Asian couples and what can we learn from the clinical case studies?

Objectives

- To introduce readers to the continuity and variations in interpersonal attachment from infancy (with caregivers) to adulthood (romantic partners)
- To review attachment styles in adulthood and how they present in romantic relationships
- To highlight key theoretical models relevant to interventions with couples that focus on attachment themes, interpersonal relational style and emotional regulation
- To synthesise literature from various evidence-based models and studies across the globe that offer interventions to distressed couples and note key measurement tools, sample characteristics and relational outcomes in these populations

- To provide clinical evidence of attachment-informed psychotherapy with South-Asian clients

Methodology

We carried out a rapid review of relevant studies focusing on key word searches across google scholar and EBSCO host search engines with search terms that included "attachment", "intergenerational" "couples therapy" and "relational distress". Rapid reviews are literature reviews conducted systematically within a limited time frame and with specific databases [1]. We addressed the chapter objectives by drawing insights from two sources: synthesising information from studies matrixed during the literature review and clinical case notes from three therapists who work with couples using intergenerational attachment and relational assessments as well as interventions (MI, MP and SV). The matrix to tabulate studies included variables such as sample demographics, location (country), therapist demographics, key variables, measurements used and key findings. For the clinical case studies, each case was written up in a similar format by each of the therapists' vis-a-vis: (1) presenting concerns, (2) intergenerational assessment and relational cycle identification, (3) relational-focused and strengths-based interventions and strategies utilised to reduce distress and meet couples' therapeutic goals. The two sections are presented sequentially in the chapter.

2. Role of Internal Working Models (IWM) and Mutual Regulations Model (MRM) in attachment

Developmentally, attachment serves a survival function in babies; whereby babies rely on a consistent caregiver to meet their needs and protect them from threat or harm. The quality of these early interactions of infants and children with their caregivers shapes their subsequent and later psychological and interpersonal interactions in life [7]. This occurs through the development of the infant's internal working model; mental representations of the self and others [8, 9]. With a sensitive and responsive caregiver, infants develop a working model of others as available and themselves as worthy of care. With an inconsistent or rejecting caregiver, infants may develop a model of others as unavailable and themselves as unworthy of care. The internal working model serves a predictive purpose to imagine how a caregiver will behave and thus hold expectations or plan one's own actions in response [10, 11]. According to Bowlby [10], gradually the internal working model (IWM) representations become the property of the child and are carried into adulthood and guide how individuals attend to, interpret, and behave in close relationships [11]. Emotions and emotional communications between an infant and caregiver play a critical role in the evaluative process, shaping the infant's internal working model as well as defining goals and developmental pathways [5, 12]. Interactional behaviours of the infant, such as, looking away or looking at an object serves a self-directed or other-directed, emotional regulatory biophysiological purpose for the infant [13]. When parents are sensitive to these emotional and behavioural indicators and respond appropriately, the infant successfully attains the goal and experiences a state of positive emotion. On the contrary, when caregivers fail to respond appropriately, the infant fails to meet interactive goals and this evaluative process leads to negative emotions [12].

Tronick's mutual regulation model [12] revolutionised the understanding of reciprocal and mutually regulated systems of affective coordination in the infant-caregiver dyad [14]. For example, Tronick's Still Face (S-F) Paradigm [14] experiment, demonstrated the mismatched interactions and its effect on the infant. In this experiment, the infant and caregiver engage with each other (emotionally and physically) and after a period of engagement, the caregiver is asked to present a neutral poker face or the still-faced expression and disengage from any conversation or physical contact with the infant. This period of disengagement is followed by a period of reunion, where the caregiver reengages with the infant. During the period of disengagement, the infant tries diverse affective repairs to engage the still-faced caregiver. The infant's failure to repair the emotional engagement with the caregiver induces stress, negative emotions (anger, protests, frustration, and sadness) and creates a mismatch [14]. However, in the reunion phase, when the caregiver re-engages and the infant responds with positive emotions, the parent's regulatory role is established, and the affective mismatch is repaired successfully. However, longer duration of infant-caregiver dyadic mismatch creates developmental pathways for psychopathology and relational distress [14, 15].

In depressed mother-infant dyads, the disengagement and interactions from caregivers limits the infant's ability to transform negative affect to positive, and is detrimental to the mental health of the infant [12]. Several researchers have tested the MRM model, for instance, Egmose and colleagues [16] conducted a comparative study on mutual regulation through touching behaviours in two sets of dyads (24 postpartum depressed mother-infant dyads, and 47 non-clinical mother-infant dyads). They found that mothers use different touching behaviours to regulate infant's negative versus positive facial affect and infants respond with negative versus positive affect to different maternal touching behaviours too. Typically, caregiving maternal touch (parent behaviour displayed by adjusting the infant's seat or wiping their mouth) are used to regulate infants' negative facial affect whereas playful touch (such as, tickling, jiggling, and large movements with the arms) are used to enhance positive affect. Moreover, infants were more likely to demonstrate positive affect due to a playful maternal touch and decrease in negative affect as a result of caregiving maternal touch [16]. Contrary to previous findings that depressed mothers do not engage with their infants, mothers with postpartum depression, in this study, used affectionate touch (such as, patting, nuzzling, kissing, stroking or caressing) to reduce negative infant facial affect as compared to non-clinical mothers [16].

Consequently, developmental pathways are shaped by the infant's moment-by-moment meaning-making process in the mutually regulating dyadic relational system. Thereby, increasing the emotional and coping capacities of the infant and creating coherence in the dyadic system through repeated reparations [12, 14, 15]. This also creates diversity and complexity in the infant's experiences to successfully self-regulate and use the other (the caregiver) as a regulatory mechanism, thereby shaping the infant's ability to transform negative to positive emotions and influencing their internal working model of relationships [12, 15, 16]. However, repeated failed affective reparations leads to limited exposure to diverse experiences of reparation and lack of coherence in the infant-caregiver dyadic emotional communication [12, 15]. Recent studies have extended the understanding of mutual regulation models. The dynamic interactional intersubjective experience of knowing to be with each other and ways to repair or work things out together results in an implicit procedural knowledge, a mental representation of implicit relational knowing (IRK) [13]. Banella and Tronick [17] found evidence of UIRK in 11-month-olds as compared to 6-month-olds. This developmental change is incorporated in the memory in the form of two types of implicit knowing- relational and procedural understanding of relating. Thus, the dyadic relationship paves the way for unique patterns of relational knowing (UIRK) through mutual co-creation of meaning-making, regulation of affect and interactional understanding from the repetitive interactions and repairs at various times and contexts of daily living. Hence, the co-creation of the mutually coordinated reciprocity, whether coherent, complex or messy, is unique in infant-caregiver relationships and happens in everyday moment-by-moment interactions with the caregiver [17, 18] and becomes a part of the implicit psychobiological memory process [18]. Thereby, the unique implicit relational knowing (UIRK) [17, 18] plays a crucial role in formative relationships and influences how the infant feels about self and others in future relationships [18].

3. Attachment patterns in infancy, adolescence and adulthood

Internal working models and attachment patterns are also subject to intergenerational transmission and parenting responses [19]. In infant-parent relationships, they guide a parent's behaviour towards the infant, and, as a result, influence the infant's own developing internal working model [20–23]. A parent with a secure and consistent internal working model is more likely to interpret their infant's attachment signals appropriately, whereas a parent with an insecure internal working model is less likely to do so [24–27]. Research has demonstrated that mothers with unresolved trauma tend to have infants who display profoundly disorganised attachment [28–30]. A meta-analysis reviewing 661 mother-infant dyads found a 75% match of secure/insecure attachment classifications [31]. Similarly, findings from another study of grandmother-mother–child dyads suggested continuity of attachment patterns across three generations [32]. Thus, these attachment behaviours and dyadic interactions with caregivers develop into more enduring, permanent attachment styles in adulthood.

Ainsworth and colleagues [33] studied individual differences in attachment patterns and initially distinguished between three types of attachment in infancy: secure, anxious, and avoidant, based on the strange situation study of infant-mother interactions. Securely attached infants became upset when the mother left the room and when she returned, they actively sought their mothers and were easily comforted by them. For those infants indicating anxious attachment, they became distressed upon separation and had a difficult time being soothed during reunion. They possibly experienced uncertainty about love from their attachment figure. For infants demonstrating avoidant attachment, they appeared to be mildly distressed during separation and actively avoided their mothers upon reunion, appearing self-reliant. In later years, Main and Solomon [34, 35] added the disorganised attachment style, referring to children who have no predictable pattern of attachment behaviours. They viewed their caregiver as a source of both comfort and fear, leading to conflicting behaviours. Attachment models developed in infancy are carried throughout later years as models of connection and disconnection. They can be transferred into adult relationships [36, 37] and directly influence the quality of peer relations [38]. In teenagers and young adults, secure attachment, that takes the shape of emotional availability from caregivers, helps to form a developing worldview, build a sense of self and determines peer interactions and MH (mental health) outcomes [39]. Additionally, adolescents with secure attachment reported ease in seeking and providing support as well as finding a space among peers where they felt safe. They're able to integrate their past attachment experiences favourably and present a more developed concept of friendship. Greater insecurity to parents and peers in adolescence predicted a more anxious romantic attachment style and greater use of emotion-oriented strategies in adulthood. Avoidant attachment style was related to less support-seeking and greater isolation and the presentation of mental health concerns like depression in adult life [40]. Adolescents with ambivalent attachment struggle with managing conflict and experience intense reactions in their close relationships. Adolescents with avoidant attachment tend to avoid emotional engagement, demonstrated through coldness or distance with peers, have more interpersonal conflict and hold low expectations of what friendships mean [41, 42].

Moreover, attachment in infant-caregiver and partner relationships are unique and significantly impact the physical and psychological wellbeing of the dyads. Attachment in partner relationships is also defined as pair-bond attachments and can be compared with infant-caregiver relationship as both trigger the same hormonal and neurophysiological mechanism [43, 44]. Bartholomew and Horowitz [45] categorised adult attachment into four styles emerging from two underlying dimensions: anxiety (indicated by the extent to which individuals worry about abandonment and rejection; and avoidance (concerning the extent to which individuals limit intimacy with others). The four attachment styles are secure, preoccupied, dismissive-avoidant and fearful-avoidant. Secure attachment is characterised by low anxiety and low avoidance. Individuals have a positive model of the self as worthy of love and others as generally accepting and responsive. A preoccupied attachment style is characterised by high anxiety and low avoidance. These individuals harbour a negative model of the self as unworthy of love and thus worry about losing their partners and remain vigilant to signs their partners might be pulling away from them. To prevent this, they tend to use hyperactivating strategies to get closer to their partners to feel secure. They desire to merge with the other, expect partners to fill their needs and may be threatened by their partner's autonomy, leading to resentment and disappointment. A dismissing-avoidant style is characterised by low anxiety and high avoidance, manifesting as discomfort with intimacy and closeness in relationships. Individuals may hold a negative evaluation of others as clingy, needy and dependent. They strive to create and maintain independence, control and autonomy in their relationships because they may believe that to seek proximity is not possible or undesirable. Finally, a fearful-avoidant attachment style is characterised by both high anxiety and avoidance. These individuals desire closeness with others but fear rejection. They maintain a distance as a means to protect themselves. These four attachment styles provide a window into the way individuals relate to those close to them [45].

4. Attachment patterns in adult romantic relationships

Attachment patterns are also used to negotiate interactions with romantic partners. Hazan and Shaver [46] observed a number of parallels between infant-parent attachments and romantic relationships, including a desire to be in physical proximity to the other; seeking the other when distressed, scared or ill; and using the other as a secure base from which to explore the world. In their study, secure adults described their romantic relationships as happy, friendly, and trusting, emphasised their ability to support and accept their partner despite their faults, and had relationships that tended to last longer than both individuals with insecure attachments. More recently, attachment styles are often represented in a two-dimensional space defined by attachment avoidance and attachment anxiety [21, 45]. Bartholomew and Horowitz [45] categorised adult attachment into four styles emerging from two underlying dimensions: anxiety (indicated by the extent to which individuals worry about abandonment and rejection; and avoidance (concerning the extent to which individuals limit intimacy with others). The four attachment styles are secure, preoccupied, dismissive-avoidant and fearful-avoidant. Secure attachment is characterised by low anxiety and low avoidance. Individuals have a positive model of the self as worthy of love and others as generally accepting and responsive. A preoccupied attachment style is characterised by high anxiety and low avoidance. These individuals harbour a negative model of the self as unworthy of love and thus worry about losing their partners and remain vigilant to signs their partners might be pulling away from them. Such individuals tend to be preoccupied with issues surrounding their partner's predictability, dependability and trustworthiness [47, 48]. They tend to question their worth, worry about losing their partner and remain vigilant to signs their partner might be pulling away from them. The relationship becomes a significant focus of their lives, on which they place unrealistically high expectations [49]. They may be threatened by their partner's autonomy, leading to resentment and ambivalence. To prevent this, they tend to use hyperactivating strategies to get closer to their partners to feel secure. They desire to merge with the other, expect partners to fill their needs and may be threatened by their partner's autonomy, leading to resentment and disappointment. A dismissing-avoidant style is characterised by low anxiety and high avoidance, manifesting as discomfort with intimacy and closeness in relationships. These individuals may hold a negative evaluation of others as clingy, needy and dependent. They strive to create and maintain independence, control and autonomy in their relationships because they may believe that to seek proximity is not possible or undesirable. Individuals expressing avoidant attachment tend to be pre-eminently concerned about avoiding excessive intimacy and commitment in relationships. They find it difficult to trust others and prefer to maintain an emotional distance. In their romantic relationships they may be mistrustful and think of the relationship as emotionally demanding. They strive to create and maintain independence, control and autonomy in their relationships and evaluate their partners as needy, clingy or dependent. Avoidant partners use de-activating strategies to downplay attachment-related threats and deny attachment needs. They become defensive, underestimate the negativity of partners' messages, engage in physical and emotional withdrawal and reduce expressions of support; these behaviours often frustrate partners [50]. Finally, a fearful-avoidant attachment style is characterised by both high anxiety and avoidance. These individuals desire closeness with others but fear rejection. They maintain a distance as a means to protect themselves. These individuals are found to be more hostile and distressed during conflict-discussions, and perceive their relationships more negatively afterwards. They tend to respond to conflict with physiological arousal and hyperactivating behaviours, designed to force partners to provide more attention and support. This egocentric stance involves neglecting a partner's needs and engaging in blame and coercion. These tactics often alienate partners, creating ongoing distress. These four attachment styles provide a window into the way most individuals relate to those close to them [45].

The different insecure attachment styles are related to less positive romantic relationships in adulthood. The relationships are characterised by less interdependence, trust, commitment and satisfaction, as well as greater relational jealousy and perceived intrusiveness from the romantic partner [51, 52]. Both an anxious and avoidant attachment style are considered risk factors for the expression of aggression towards one's partner [53]. A meta-analysis of anxious and avoidant attachment styles in romantic relationships indicated that both styles have detrimental effects on physical, emotional, cognitive and behavioural aspects of romantic relationships, with attachment avoidance being more detrimental to relationship satisfaction, connectedness and support while attachment anxiousness was associated with greater relational conflicts [47, 54]. Furthermore, preoccupied, dismissive-avoidant and fearful-avoidant attachment styles when present in both partners lead to high levels of romantic disengagement [55, 56]. Conversely, secure attachments are stated to be at the core of close, fulfilling relationships. These secure relationships provide individuals with a safe haven and secure base during threatening or distressful situations [5, 57, 58]. These relationships are also characterised by greater longevity, trust, commitment, and interdependence [59, 60]. Kobak and Hazan [61] observed that secure partners engaged in more constructive problem-solving interactions than insecure partners and found significant associations between attachment security and marital satisfaction.

5. Theoretical frameworks

5.1 Interpersonal theories

Drawing on interpersonal theories of personality, Bartholomew [62] noted that individuals tend to select social partners who sustain their initial dispositions (i.e., working models). Avoidant adults may choose ambivalent partners whose dependence confirms their expectations of relationships. Similarly, an ambivalent person faced with an avoidant partner receives confirmation of their working model of relationships in which others are reluctant to get close and unwilling to commit to a relationship. So, in a way, each attachment style is drawn to re-enact a familiar script over and over again [63, 64]. Secure adults are less likely to select partners who either avoid or are preoccupied with intimacy. They would opt for secure partners who share and confirm their comfort in close relationships [65, 66]. Attachment styles may be an important dimension by which individuals choose their marital partners.

5.2 Social learning theory

Social learning theories suggest that communication and conflict resolution strategies individuals bring into the relationship are learned in the family-of-origin [67, 68]. Consistent with this theory, studies have found that family-of-origin problems were associated with poorer communication skills, expression of negative affect, lack of openness, greater avoidance behaviours and less willingness to negotiate [69, 70]. Additionally, attachment behaviours (accessibility, responsiveness, and engagement) significantly mediated the relationship between family-of-origin problems and communication skills. Wampler et al. [69] found that individuals who reported lack of attachment security intergenerationally are more likely to express negative affect, lack of openness, more avoidance and, less willingness to negotiate with their partner. Studies have also focused on the quality of the participants' parents' relationship with each other, and when individuals perceived poor marital relations in the family-of-origin, it negatively affected their attributions about their partner's communication and perceived emotional connection [71, 72].

5.3 Attachment theory

More broadly, attachment theory is recognised as one of the most important frameworks for understanding romantic relationships [73] and its formation and success [70]. Insecurely attached partners encounter fears of closeness, feelings of jealousy, attitudes of distrust and heightened overall relational distress [74]. When presenting in couples therapy, they often raise behavioural and emotional concerns around not being prioritised enough or being ignored by their partner, feeling overwhelmed by partners' feelings, experiencing financial and logistical difficulties or difficulties navigating relationships outside of the couple unit like parents, children and so on [75, 76]. When individuals begin to distrust their partner's accessibility, responsiveness and engagement, they withdraw from each other. This weakens the relationship, further exacerbating the partners' fears and anxieties and worsening their mental health [77–79]. Oftentimes, these concerns manifest as relational mistrust, lack of quality time spent together, high levels of conflict, blaming or withdrawal from one partner and a host of other poor adaptations or outcomes. This leaves individuals more vulnerable and exposed to stress and developing mental health concerns [80] including generalised anxiety, depression and symptoms of psychosis [81–84].

Numerous studies have found strong empirical support for differences in relationship satisfaction, psychological well-being (e.g., self-esteem, depression) and childhood experiences as a function of secure, avoidant, and ambivalent attachment styles in adulthood [45, 85, 86]. While longitudinal studies have provided the strongest evidence for the continuity of attachment styles from childhood to adulthood [87–89], other research studies have shown that attachments are subject to change based on new experiences and relationship environments [21, 45, 60, 90]. This provides an opportunity for intervention research to explore and evaluate how relational, attachment-focused interventions might serve as mechanisms of positive change for insecure attachment styles. Studies have shown that clinical interventions can be effective in shifting people's attachment anxiety and avoidance. For example, asking people to reflect on fostering security in their relationships and/or experiences appears to cause them to behave more securely. They're able to exhibit greater empathetic, creative and responsive behaviours [91–95]. Interventions that are repeatedly administered, may be able to change people's enduring trait level anxiety and avoidance, with effects on relationship functioning and wellbeing [96, 97]. Furthermore, looking at how family-of-origin experiences spill out into interactional patterns with one's spouse may be one way to improve marital communication. This provides an optimistic view of relationships for those who have experienced negative family-of-origin experiences including high family conflict, violence, hostility and parental divorce [70].

Therefore, models and therapies with a relational focus- which emphasises holding awareness of the self, other and the relationship, might be one approach to help re-engage couples, reaffirm affection between romantic partners as well as ultimately help sustain intimacy and satisfaction [56]. Furthermore, when the emotions and motivations of romantic partners are framed as their expressed need, there is a greater scope to look at problematic interactional cycles and find scope for change through new experiences [98, 99]. The skills learned in therapy including positive communication and healthy conflict resolution are also strongly associated with greater marital satisfaction [99].

6. Efficacy studies from intervention models

To better understand the mechanisms of adult attachment, various empirically supported treatments for couples have been developed and tested in the last few decades [100–105]. The most prominent evidence base is for attachment-focused and communication enhancing models including emotionally focused couples therapy (EFcT), integrative behavioural couples therapy (IBCT) and the Gottman method. These models view presenting problems as symptoms of struggles with interpersonal effectiveness and communication, as a result of insecure attachments.

Several different therapeutic modalities have been measured against one another to assess the impact on relational outcomes. Byrne et al. [106] studied the efficacy of behavioural couples therapy and emotionally focused couples therapy with distressed couples. Across 20 studies (13 IBCT and 7 EFcT), they found that IBCT fares better than 83% and EFcT 89% of untreated couples and these gains were maintained at a 2-year follow up. Ahmadi et al. [107] and Havaasi et al. [105] found that EFcT and Gottman couple therapy methods reduced marital burnout and changed conflict resolution styles ($P < 0.05$), with EFcT being more effective. In EFcT specifically, increasing awareness of primary and secondary emotions and encouraging the partner who typically takes a blaming/critical stance to express their attachment needs and fears (blamer-softening), were responsible for facilitating further decreases in couples' attachment insecurity and relationship distress [108, 109]. This change occurs through an increase in both partners' level of engagement during therapy, especially those who are classified with avoidant attachment styles, especially men who have higher disengagement scores especially when paired with anxiously attached partners [56]. Especially men higher on attachment avoidance reported greater romantic disengagement at follow-up. Moser et al. [110] found that there were measured decreases in attachment avoidance and attachment anxiety (following blamer softening sessions) and an overall increase in relational satisfaction upon completion of EFcT. Therefore, changes in relationship-specific attachment anxiety, secure attachment behaviours and relationship functioning may be long-lasting and continue to improve in the years following therapy for those couples who engaged in and completed EFcT [104].

The most common measures used to gather data on attachment styles are the Experience in Close Relationships (ECR), the Adult Attachment Scale (AAS), the Adult Attachment Interview (AAI) and the Brief Accessibility Responsiveness and Engagement Scale (BARE). While these measures attempt to record the same aspects of functioning in close relationships, they predict outcomes captured at different developmental stages resulting in low convergence between measures [21].Other relational and functional measures across studies have been checking relationship satisfaction via the Dyadic Adjustment Scale (DAS), the Relate Scale of Family Quality and Family Communication, Pine's measure for Burnout, Rahim Organizational Conflict Inventory (ROCI) for conflict resolution, Romantic Disengagement Scale (RDS), the relational Q-sort, The Secure Base Scoring System (SBSS) and Difficulties in Emotional Regulation Scale (DERS) for emotional regulation.

Across studies, EFcT, which focuses on improving attachment styles and de-escalating conflict, has been seen as an effective intervention for all of the above outcomes. Specifically, EFcT has been found across studies to improve relationship satisfaction between partners and increase attunement and responsive behaviours, characteristic of secure attachment and reduced attachment anxiety and/or avoidance between partners [111, 112]. Benson et al. [113] concluded that changes in attachment style (especially attachment anxiety) and marital satisfaction work concurrently over the course of therapy. EFcT has also been found effective for a number of populations expressing a variety of concerns including cancer care [114], PTSD [115], depression in one of the romantic partners [116], spousal abuse [117] and infertility [118]. EFcT and Gottman have also been tested cross-culturally with promising findings in Iran, Ireland, Israel, Taiwan and Thailand [72, 107, 119–121]. However, there are drawbacks to these findings. A significant limitation is that a majority of these studies are tested in North America and by teams led by or advised by the model developers which leads to allegiance effects and lack of cultural transferability [119]. In terms of participants, most studies have also been conducted with heterosexual, married couples in their middle age (late 30s to mid-40s). Additionally, in several studies, the therapists training and identities have not been considered as a co-variant factor and data has been collected by largely using self-report measures. In our contribution, we aim to expand the research on attachment by providing more experiential narratives through therapeutic case vignettes across age groups, genders and sexuality orientations.

7. Case studies

We have used Benson et al.'s framework [122] while looking into the cases. He proposed that there are five common evidence-based factors or principles to guide interventions with couples experiencing relationship distress. They are: (1) altering the couple's view of the presenting problem to be more objective, adult-focused problems, (2) decreasing emotion-driven, dysfunctional behaviour; (3) eliciting emotion-based, avoided, private behaviour; (4) increasing constructive communication patterns; and (5) promoting strengths and reinforcing gains.

7.1 Case study 1

Ali and Samara are a young couple in their late 20s. Ali works in the Indian armed forces and is posted in a different location every few years while Samara lives in the national capital of India- New Delhi. They have known each other since high school and began their relationship as friends. Ali had been in love with Samara for years but they only began dating one another in 2019 and subsequently got married in 2021. They presented to therapy raising concerns of a lack of adjustment to each other's needs post marriage, divergent opinions in decision making, feeling dissatisfied in their relationship and feeling unsure about their future together.

7.1.1 Initial sessions and assessment

A total of 14 sessions were conducted with the therapist (*MI, first author*). The first few sessions involved a systemic assessment of their relationship history, identifying other key stakeholders (parents, siblings and friends) as well as more recent contextual issues (arguments about relationships with respective families-of-origin, Samara's recent abortion, individual career plans, finances and heightened emotional interactions during conflicts). The plan for attachment-oriented emotionally focused couples therapy as a treatment format was shared after discussing hopes for their relationship and setting goals in therapy. As per EFcT, a few sessions explored their cycle of conflict and increasing awareness to help de-escalate future conflict. Next, attachment styles were explored. This was obtained through individual sessions with each partner where an attachment narrative was drawn, their understanding around their attachment styles and resultant emotions were deepened. Finally, partners were brought back together for joint sessions to address injuries in their attachment, increase their sense of longing for support and cohesion along with deliberating on possible goals for the future.

7.1.2 Relational conflict cycle

The relational conflicts for Samara and Ali seemed to originate with them wanting to plan out certain crucial life priorities. For Samara, this included immediately being in an independent home of their own where Ali could visit and spend time when he was not at a posting in the armed forces. For Ali, this included buying a car and financial planning for a future home. Furthermore, individual needs also came to the fore. Samara wished to pursue higher studies in a doctorate abroad and Ali expressed exhaustion around his current posting and wished for further training and self-development between his postings. This would often lead to issues about whose needs to prioritise, lack of time for each other and continuing disagreements. Samara would get agitated and display heightened emotions, that caused Ali to shut down. Repetitive pleas from Samara to solve their conflicts led to Ali withdrawing further or having anger outbursts that traumatised Samara and reminded her of how she felt in her own family. Ali would feel embarrassed by his behaviour and withdraw from her or distract himself instead of connecting with her when she was in this hurt state.

7.1.3 Intergenerational attachment history of both partners

Samara- In individual sessions, her relationships within her family-of-origin were explored. It came to light that Samara had taken on the role of a caretaker for her mother and felt parentified because her mother struggles with chronic physical and mental health issues, including diabetes and bipolar disorder. As a result, she had not felt like she could lean on her mother or rely on her to meet her emotional needs. Samara's father also worked in the armed forces and would spend a lot of time away from the family. When he was home, he was also a stickler for discipline, schedule and financial control. Samara often felt that she did not get enough pocket money or allowances from her parents. As a result, she began to do part-time jobs at the age of 16. This perceived lack of importance or having low value to her parents may have resulted in Samara's anxious-preoccupied attachment style, and is reflected in her relationship with Ali, especially given their long-distance relationship. In individual sessions, MI deepened her emotions around her anxieties for finances, which also manifested in her relationship with Ali, when he would not send her the house rental allowance payments on time or wanted to buy a car that was beyond their means. In her attachment style with Ali, she identified how she would make demands or pleas for her emotions to be validated during difficult times (i.e., the abortion or when there was forcefulness from his parents about having a baby) and for her needs to be met but when disregarded she became blaming, hopeless and disengaged, feeling like he did not care for her or that she was of no value to him.

Ali- In individual sessions with Ali, an exploration of his intergenerational attachment history revealed that he did not feel close to either of his parents and had no other significant caregivers that he relied on during his early years. Ali changed homes and schools frequently due to his father's job and was physically punished at home and in school for low academic performance. He faced adjustment issues and was bullied by his peers due to his accent, physical appearance and shy personality. On one occasion, he was described to have been bullied badly by his peers and was held accountable for something he did not do. He lost his sense of trust and reliance on his parents being there for him. The parents followed the advice of his school principal and he was suspended for a few weeks. The topic was never discussed in his family and Ali felt he had been punished and made invisible. The above factors may have laid the foundation for his tendency to withdraw from others and his avoidant attachment style.

Through individual sessions, MI deepened his emotions and experiences around being bullied, feeling like an outcast and his subsequent mental health concerns. He discussed that his mental health concerns of depression and lack of focus and concentration on academic goals became a source of great embarrassment in his family and till date, he withholds sharing his struggles in the armed forces with his parents and Samara. He attempts to protect Samara from his parent's style of relating to the couple which includes high expectations, low levels of attunement and an environment of subservience to their advice. As a result, Samara feels tentative around his family and that he is constantly hiding things from her. His difficulty with opening up to her emotionally also exacerbates her insecurities about herself and increases her demands for attention, validation and care.

7.1.4 Interventions based on attachment needs

Bringing them back together in joint sessions was important but metaphorically also helped them turn towards each other to address attachment wounds and explore the significant ruptures in their relationship, instead of turning away and feeling isolated.

7.1.5 Softening the anxious partner

T: So, Samara, you had brought up how hurt you felt by Ali when you could not talk about the abortion and the argument you both had about his parents' reaction that you should have the baby. This was a major moment of pain for you. Can you share this with Ali and give him a chance to understand better this time around?

S: I basically felt that he deferred to them when they were trying to make a decision about my body. It was dehumanising and it felt like I was on my own in the world, the same way I felt when I was younger.

A: I am truly sorry for making you feel that way. It was a moment of panic for me too but I should have not shut down and instead been there for you, for us. I often get intimidated by my parents and fear disappointing them- with my academics, my career, my personal choices. It's something I need to work on.

7.1.6 Re-engaging the avoidant partner

T: Ali, we spoke about your experiences of being bullied and how that impacted your well-being and functioning. It sounds like this happens to you when Samara is upset and blames you. In these situations, you feel that she, just like your parents, are not on your side and that you are being attacked or picked on. Can you share more on this with her?

A: Yes. I feel that Samara is also trying to embarrass me or put me down. I tend to feel like everything is my fault or that I am the failure and I shut you out with silent treatment. I pull away from you (*use of distancing strategies).*

T: What do you need from Samara during these times?

A: To make space for my feelings and to notice that I am holding back to avoid more fights with her, that I want peace with her.

T: Samara, did you know that Ali tries to pull away so you fight less?

S: I guess I had realised that it was his way of diffusing the situation but I am only now realising it comes at a cost to him.

T: How does this feel for you Samara, when Ali pulls away?

S: I feel like I have been abandoned by him and I mean nothing to him (*low self-worth emerges*). I get scared that he will leave me.

T: Ali, were you aware of how your actions impacted her emotionally and that she is scared to lose you? (*Creating space for longing and re-connection).*

A: I did not and would not ever want her to feel that way. I was simply trying to keep her away from my own confusions about my career so she would not get concerned about our future.

7.1.7 Designing and building a future together

Towards the end of therapy, goals were discussed in a mutual and reciprocal way. They included dividing finances, supporting each other to achieve individual milestones and plan career trajectories and drawing healthy boundaries between themselves and others, especially the involvement of his parents in decisions like child-bearing, investments, etc. Ali shared with Samara that he did not see himself working in the armed forces in the longer-term. He would like to quit in the next few years to explore a career associated with his true passion, golf. We also discussed how that would potentially help them chart out a path which considered both partners wishes. We also spoke about how Ali could be flexible in his posting based on where Samara would pursue her PhD, and reduce the number of years continuing a long-distance relationship. They ended therapy with the motivation to be more attuned to each other, have empathy for their respective attachment styles and to further the skills they acquired during therapy to communicate more cohesively.

7.2 Case study 2

Priya and Raman are in their mid-40s. They have been in a relationship for 20 years and married for 15 years. Priya wants to seek couples therapy as she and Raman have become distant from each other and their marriage lacks intimacy. They hardly share their feelings with each other, and when they do it escalates into a major conflict with Raman distancing himself and Priya feeling overwhelmed and hurt in the relationship. For Priya, if their present status quo is maintained, she can no longer see herself in a marriage with Raman. Although Raman did not want counselling, he agreed to try couples therapy on Priya's insistence. He understands that if he does not participate, Priya will file for divorce. He does not want to start over again in life at this age and they have a daughter to think about. Therefore, he has agreed to therapy. Both agreed that their relationship has reached a level of stagnancy after years of being together. They both identified issues of trust, intimacy and stagnancy in their relationship.

7.2.1 Relational conflict cycle

A total of 24 sessions were conducted with the therapist (*MP, second author*). Initial sessions with the couple revealed that the major conflict in their marital relationship was the pattern of distancing and closeness, lack of trust and not feeling valued in the relationship. Raman prefers to maintain his emotional independence and does not like sharing, and he finds Priya very clingy and intrusive. Individual sessions with Priya revealed her challenges in her marital relationship.

Priya: According to Priya, they had a greater degree of physical, emotional and intellectual closeness in the first few years of their life together. Though Raman was the one who wanted to be romantically involved with her, she was the one who proposed marriage after a few years of dating him. She shared that he got married because of her insistence on marriage. They enjoyed each other's company, the intellectual conversations, wit and passion. They identified themselves as a modern, liberal and egalitarian couple. Neither wanted kids at that point. However, 6 years into their relationship, Priya spoke about her desire to be a mother. They had a daughter 6 years into their marriage. Both were working professionals with demanding jobs. Priya ended up making a lot of sacrifices at her workplace to raise their daughter, as Raman would travel a lot. She had to become involved and sometimes it seemed that she was giving too much in the relationship as a parent and partner and did not feel valued. Though she perceived her sexual relationship as good, what she missed was emotional closeness and physical demonstration of love and intimacy such as holding hands, hugging and sharing feelings and thoughts with her. Sometimes, she did not understand what went on in Raman's mind; he does not disclose. Raman is social, approachable, amicable, witty, attractive, friendly, and has an intellectual command over many subjects but he is very private about his own feelings and avoids personal disclosure. Both have many friends from the same and opposite sex and it previously never bothered them. However, Priya feels that his female friends behave inappropriately with him, such as clinging to him or caressing his arms and he does not stop them. Such displays of intimacy aren't shared with her and he also does not express pleasure when she initiates such displays of intimacy. She struggles with trust and level of intimacy in their relationship.

Raman: According to Raman, they were happy for a while and then Priya insisted on having a child and Raman conceded. He found Priya to be too demanding and he did not want to upset their relationship. He also loved her; however, he never asked or expected her to make sacrifices in her career. They were both working professionals and had child care at home and also received support from their in-laws. Though Raman was a hands-on father and as parents they worked well together, in parenting their daughter, Priya took most of the decisions about their daughter. Raman loves his daughter dearly and they get along well. According to him, both spend quality time with their daughter. If one of them is travelling, the other takes care of their daughter. Raman too expressed problems with intimacy. He found it challenging to express love as a married couple after being in a relationship for such a long time. It seems childish to hold hands, hug each other like in Bollywood or Hollywood movies. They both socialise a lot, and have common friends. He mentioned that Priya is possessive and there are trust issues in their relationship along with intimacy. Raman mentioned that if they are at a party, and any of their female friends pull him onto the dance floor or rub his shoulder, Priya gets upset. He shared that he does not show fondness, attention or initiative with another woman. On his part, he finds it rude to stop some women when they request him for a dance or hug him. After all, these are their common friends. According to him, he has been faithful to Priya and has not had any relationship outside his marriage. He described not having any intention to jeopardise his relationship. However, Priya lacks trust in their relationship.

7.2.2 Intergenerational attachment history of both partners

A genogram provided an intergenerational narrative of the family relationship history and the narratives of closeness and distance in the couple's relationship. Priya's parents had a conventional marriage. Her mother was warm and loving and her father was the stern disciplinarian and the head of the family. She tried to live up to the expectations of her parents, especially her father. She seeks his validation, respect and appreciation. However, they also have different perspectives, opinions, choices, and disagree very often with each other. Her father shuts down when they argue, and this behaviour irritates her. Therefore, at times she wants closeness with her father, and sometimes, she does not. She is more emotionally invested in her relationship with her father; however, he does not understand, appreciate or reciprocate as per her expectations. She reported a similar pattern of communication and relationship narratives with Raman.

Raman, on the other hand, had a different intergenerational narrative. His parents were very reserved and quiet. His parents barely argued with each other and never raised their voice to express their displeasure. They valued composure, calmness, and intellectual pursuits. Some physical demonstrations of love were shown by his mother; however, his father maintained a very strict demeanour. Raman remembered himself as a rebellious child, getting into conflicts with his father. However, his father never raised his voice even when he expressed his displeasures. His family pursued intelligent discussions rather than emotional and physical displays of love during family time. Raman shared that as a child he may have wanted his parents' validation or appreciation but he let go of these expectations a long time ago. He does not express or share his feelings with Priya and others, similar to how his family behaved.

The mismatch in the communication emerged from for both Priya and Raman's narrative. Priya's revelation shows that she has anxious attachment, whereas Raman displays avoidant attachment in their relationship history. Finally, an assessment of the patterns of conflict in the couple's relationship revealed that Raman withdraws from intimacy, whereas Priya pursues physical and emotional intimacy. They repeat the distance-pursuer patterns of communication where the wife demands and the husband withdraws from connection in their relationship.

7.2.3 Interventions based on Gottman Method Couple Therapy

The Gottman Method Couple Therapy guides the therapist to focus on the initial conjoint and individual session to understand the positives and the negatives in the relationship and the shared meaning making process in the couple relationship. In addition, the individual sessions provide an understanding of the individual partner's history of relationship with the parents and the parental relationship [123]. The therapist also works with the couple to identify the patterns of conflict (such as the four horsemen-criticism, contempt, withdrawal and stonewalling). Interventions are designed to help the couple down-regulate negative affect, up-regulate positive affect and develop shared meaning making. Furthermore, focusing on improving the positive to negative interactions provides stability to the couple relationship [123].

7.2.4 Focusing on the positives

Both Raman and Priya agreed that intimacy has been a major conflict in their relationship and trust issues stemmed from lack of fulfilment in their relationship. However, both were able to identify certain strengths in their relationships. Both identified each other as important in their life. They agreed that they have maintained respect towards each other, even in their anger. They are not physically or verbally abusive towards each other unlike other couples in their peer group. Priya still finds Raman charming and witty and for Raman, he described Priya to be a very talented and artistic individual. They also respect each other's individuality unlike their own families. Therefore, the couple values each other as individuals in their relationship.

7.2.5 Focusing on the negatives

The therapy sessions also involved the couple identifying the disruptive patterns of communication and the associated meaning for each partner. When Priya approaches Raman for connection, whether through physical or emotional intimacy and he withdraws, she experiences hurt. She does not feel appreciated, and when he does not stop their common friend from hugging him or rubbing her hand on his face or arms, Priya feels a deep sense of rejection, jealousy, and distrust. For Priya, physical demonstration of love, such as giving her hugs, holding her hands, touching her hair and cheeks or accepting her non-sexual touch are means of staying connected and feeling secure in their relationship. For her, enjoying emotional closeness and disclosure meant that she valued and appreciated Raman. Conversely, Raman's disengagement is perceived as insulting and she feels defensive. Raman, on the other hand, viewed that as a middle-aged couple, they did not need physical demonstration of love. He did not learn to value them or express his appreciation or love to his partner in such a manner. It also helps him limit his expectations and prevents him from being vulnerable. He discussed feeling vulnerable and less secure about expressing love. It is easy for him not to expect and prefers to be independent. It minimises hurt, expectations and vulnerability. However, when Priya insists, he feels attacked and becomes defensive and withdraws from her.

7.2.6 Focusing on the shared meaning-making

The therapist facilitated the meaning-making and assisted in identifying the negative and dysfunctional patterns of communication and connection. In addition, the therapist also helped the couple assess the level of positive to negative interactions in their relationships and helped each partner listen to the other's narratives. The couple practised 'I statements' in expressing their feelings safely in-session, while the other partner listened. The couple was given homework assignments to practice healthy communication. Multiple ways of sharing were discussed, while Priya preferred verbal discussion, Raman preferred writing small notes. Examining and exploring each partner's love languages, and strengthening their positive interactions through these love languages helped the couple. Gradually, resolving the couple's conflicts included working on assignments such as listening to each other, processing each other's gripe, discussing a repair checklist and collaboratively working on a complaint] together. Raman and Priya worked on repairing their relationship by improving their communication (physical, verbal and written expression of appreciation and closeness). As a couple, Raman and Priya also came up with a shared symbol that would indicate to the other that the partner is feeling overwhelmed, devalued or hurt. This shared symbol allowed Priya to express without feeling overwhelmed, and Raman to request for space without feeling pushed. Towards the end of therapy, the couple felt confident and secure in expressing their closeness, however, they agreed that this would be a work in progress and they will continue to use the tools learnt in therapy for improving their relationship.

7.3 Case study 3

Prana and Chhavi had been in a relationship for 2 years when they came to therapy (with therapist SV, chapter contributor). Both are AFAB (Assigned Female At Birth). Prana uses she/they pronouns and Chhavi uses she/her pronouns. The therapeutic contact lasted for around 6 months. Prana works in the restaurant management space and Chhavi works in social media marketing and with ad agencies. Prana is in their late 30s and Chhavi is in their early 30s. They met in the queer space and had both just stepped out from other relationships. The two-year relationship involved feeling very connected at the beginning of the relationship, finding a lot of relief and camaraderie in each other and things moving quite fast. One year into the relationship, they started living together. However, with time, cracks started to appear. Prana had grown up with a lot of neglect in the family. She also felt a lack of closure and abandonment in previous relationships. Chhavi has always been a high achiever and lives with ADHD. She experiences high energy bursts and wants to try a lot of things. She has felt like she had to do a lot to earn basic praise from her parents. She has had partners who have sometimes been distant, while other partners have been too close and suffocating.

7.3.1 Relational conflict cycle

The presenting concern they came with was that they were having a lot of fights, and also that Chhavi wanted to try an open relationship format where she could see other people while Prana was still the primary partner. They had been to a therapist before and because the fights about open relationships and polyamory were not going anywhere, the previous therapist had asked to pause the conversation on that topic. That had improved things in the short-term. They stopped fighting and saw a slight improvement in their intimacy and communication. However, off late, the discomforts and fights started again, which they wanted to address, and also, they wanted to be able to discuss polyamory in a useful way. The therapist's understanding about this was that while polyamory may be the presenting issue, it feels like it's a metaphor for other aspects that both of them feel, abandonment vs. suffocation, and that has in some way or the other, come up in the fights.

Chhavi seemed to want more from intimate spaces, this included seeing other people but also more from Prana. This included more emotional attunement, more praise, more warmth, and in all, a lot of verbal validation. Prana on the other hand, was seeing this as betrayal and abandonment because of past experiences – neglect at the hand of parents and breakups that did not have adequate closure.

Both of them were already facing the brunt of stigma as an invisible couple in many spaces. Their parents and cis-het friends often saw them as friends and not as a couple. They were told not to tell their grandparents due to it being 'too much' and would harm the health of the older people. While Prana was out at their workplace to colleagues, Chhavi had to navigate masking her gender identity at work and home too.

The therapist used the Sue Johnson model of negative cycles to conceptualise as well as to explain to the couple, how their defences were feeding off each other. The more Prana became rigid and distant, like a punishing parent, the more Chhavi felt like having multiple partners would meet her needs. However, Prana felt that polyamory would put a lot of pressure on their relationship, be a test of trust and Prana feared that Chhavi may fall out of love. When Prana held too tight due to previous abandonment experiences, Chhavi felt more and more suffocated and started to withdraw in behaviour while withholding communication with Prana. She felt alienated as her emotional and physical needs were not being heard or met. Prana continued to disallow any changes in their relationship and then became deeply wounded every time Chhavi brought up polyamory in therapy.

7.3.2 Intergenerational attachment history of both partners

Chhavi seemed to hold an avoidant attachment style and Prana had an anxious attachment style. Prana tended to over-explain not wanting an open relationship, got really worried about losing the relationship, found it hard to focus at work and was not able to set boundaries for each partner's personal space. Chhavi, on the other hand, tended to get into alternating cycles of frustration followed by withdrawal by getting distant whenever they had a major fight or there was an expression of Prana's imagined hurt and distrust.

7.3.3 Interventions based on attachment needs

In the first few sessions, we worked on the idea of balancing adventure with domesticity (the need for safety vs. adventure as posited by Esther Perel) and they decided that while they need a good together time – it needs to be more than problem solving, to actually "being" with each other too. They also needed equally good away time so that they could come back to the relationship recharged. Chhavi and Prana tend to share a child-caregiver dynamic. Chhavi is often in need of reminders for relational care or care of their domestic life. Prana takes the caretaker role in their relationship, which has a flip side of making Chhavi feel suffocated or infantilised and Prana feeling like they are the only one being 'mature'. Inadvertently, this led to a ranking of needs in the relationship, where Chhavi's desires are viewed as shameful or needy, and infantilized and punished at times when Prana does not want to play the caretaker or gets tired of that role.

We discussed more about how these roles having become too rigid and both partners needed to shift their stance with Chhavi stepping up so that Prana does not feel like a caregiver and Prana needing to view Chhavi's needs as a personal preference in intimacy and not be condescending towards her. The therapist also shared how Prana can step back from the caregiver role and let mistakes, forgetting, etc. happen without fearing loss of control and allowing for relational learning to happen through that, if they want to avoid feeling burnout as the caregiver.

Both of them got COVID one after the other, so meeting each other and doing some of the homework discussed, became difficult. The next few sessions were spent trying to identify the concerns with polyamory as well as the concerns with current relational patterns. We spoke of conflict being normal, and using the Gottman method to repair and de-escalate. The therapy sessions focused on how to not generalise the negatives to the entire person but keep it isolated to the behaviour at hand and watch out for contempt. The therapist also discussed how the distancer-pursuer cycle can become too familiar with time but may not be helpful to relational fulfilment. They discussed a few examples of when this had happened and the outcomes. The therapeutic space was also used to discuss that it's not just about changing roles and going from pursuer to distancer or vice versa. Rather, it is about naming the uncomfortable emotions that drives that cycle – feeling fear, uncertainty, lack of love – and working with them directly. We did a few practice attempts within the session where they could talk about a concern while still staying loving towards the other, being clear about their needs and being flexible for the most suitable outcome.

After these few sessions and during the pandemic, they became irregular with sessions. The therapist had a suspicion that they were in a complacent state and the pandemic had made them numb their reactions to each other. So, they were probably back to a certain status quo, until something happens to bring the instability again. An incident followed that sparked and re-escalated their conflict. Chhavi was attracted to someone at a party and expressed romantic interest in them. When Prana saw this, they did not say anything and just began stonewalling Chhavi. They waited for Chhavi to bring it up. When she did, it led to a huge fight and they reached a stalemate again. This time, they came back to therapy admitting that they should have been more regular and committed to therapy which could also be a metaphor not just for therapy but also for being more attuned to each other, communicating better and trying to step out of older, rigid roles and patterns. Prana expressed anger and wanted polyamory off the table if they were to sustain the relationship in the future. The therapist discussed how ultimatums were not the solution and reflected on these threats being a result of intergenerational neglect from Prana's parents.

Therapy focused on Prana's pain and Chhavi responding to that rather than simply seeing Prana as rigid while she was pushing for polyamory. This helped Prana feel seen and heard. Chhavi shared that her goal was not to neglect Prana and was more an ask of expanding intimacy and sexual connection with others, in a safe way. They both spoke of different ways of spending time, bringing up sensitive topics, being emotionally present and also trying to understand each other's historical trauma over time. This would help them both see where the other was coming from and respond in the most fruitful way, rather than just speaking to defend one's position. Chhavi decided to give it 6 months to see how she feels about polyamory, and till then, both decided to give their fullest to the relationship at hand rather than focus on looming threats. If after this, Chhavi still felt like changing the format of the relationship, Prana promised to try and look at it differently rather than as a competition. They said they would look up polyamory and study it in a little more detail.

The therapist reflected on how she sometimes became a nurturer to Chhavi and the alliance became split such that Prana felt neglected. The balance was tricky and difficult and sometimes, the therapist's own parents' dysfunctional marriage would come to mind and make her feel on edge.

7.3.4 Special considerations for this population

Addressing issues in a queer relationship with AFAB partners, polyamory and commitment, issues of patriarchy/gender roles, etc. When people are socialised as girls or female children, there are certain traits that are encouraged and certain that are discouraged. Therefore, when we honour people's gender identities, this part of their upbringing cannot be ignored. Secondly, whenever someone has a marginalised identity, they have often been wounded and deprived by society and their loved ones in many ways. Their suppressed feelings the testing and justice-seeking process can often come up in close and intimate relationships, sometimes as entitlement, and at other times as issues with commitment, communication, etc. Therefore, it is important to keep the deprivation and the related repetition compulsion in mind.

Having internalised cis-heterosexual ideas, queer people too can think of monogamy as better and purer and look down on polyamory as cheating, abandonment and a way to escape seriousness and commitment. These thoughts and beliefs need to be addressed side by side as we work on what it is that ideas like these evoke.

8. Conclusion

In this chapter, we delineate the continuity of attachment from infancy to adulthood to showcase how intergenerational patterns with early caregivers may present in romantic relationships. As differing attachment styles present in romantic relationships between partners, so too emerges the scope for understanding each partner's attachment needs, increasing mutual attunement and emotional regulation. This brings into focus the scope for couples therapy. Interventions via promotive couples therapy is at the crux of developing more fulfilling relationships and increasing relational stability in couples of diverse ethnicities and genders or sexual orientations. These interventions are also applicable irrespective of marital status or length of the relationship. The efficacy studies we reviewed indicate that emotionally focused couples therapy, Gottman's therapy and integrative behavioural couples therapy are a few of the key models with shared underlying mechanisms. These mechanisms include identifying individual needs, focusing on relational strengths, shared relationship visions and fostering a lasting emotional bond between partners. The three case studies review how three separate therapists (MI, MP and SV) utilise a shared process of relational history taking and conceptualization, focusing on individual relational needs and intervening based on the above therapeutic models. Case details were modified by the therapists to protect clients' confidentiality. Through the writing of this chapter, we hope to bring more representation to diverse couples and highlight the scope of common factors, as they are implemented in relational therapies.

Acknowledgements

We sincerely thank Sadaf Vidha (SV) of Guftagu therapy for her contribution to the case studies.

Author details

Maliha Ibrahim[1*], Manjushree Palit[1] and Rhea Matthews[2]

1 OP Jindal Global University, Sonepat, India

2 Independent Practitioner, New Delhi, India

*Address all correspondence to: maliha.ibrahim89@gmail.com

References

[1] Tricco AC, Antony J, Zarin W, Strifler L, Ghassemi M, Ivory J, et al. A scoping review of rapid review methods. BMC Medicine. 2015;**13**(1):224

[2] Bowlby J. The Making and Breaking of Affectional Bonds. London: Tavistock Publication; 1979

[3] Bowlby J. Attachment and Loss, Vol. 1: Attachment. New York: Basic Books; 1969

[4] Bowlby J. Attachment and loss: Retrospect and prospect. The American Journal of Orthopsychiatry. 1982;**52**(4):664-678. DOI: 10.1111/j.1939-0025.1982.tb01456.x

[5] Bowlby J. Attachment and Loss. Vol. 2: Separation: Anxiety and Anger. New York: Basic Books; 1973

[6] Ainsworth MD, Bell SM, Stayton DJ. Individual differences in Strange-Situation behaviour of one-year-olds. In: Schaffer HR, editor. The Origins of Human Social Relations. New York: Academic Press; 1973. p. 17

[7] Feeney JA. Adult romantic attachment: Developments in the study of couple relationships. In: Cassidy J, Shraver PR, editors. Handbook of Attachment: Theory, Research, and Clinical Applications. New York: The Guilford Press; 2008. p. 456

[8] Parkes CM, Hinde JS. The Place of Attachment in Human Behaviour. London: Tavistock Publications; 1982

[9] Engels RC, Finkenauer C, Meeus W, Deković M. Parental attachment and adolescents' emotional adjustment: The associations with social skills and relational competence. Journal of Counseling Psychology. 2001;**48**:428-439. DOI: 10.1037//0022-0167.48.4.428

[10] Bowlby J. A Secure Base: Parent Child Attachment and Healthy Human Development. New York: Basic Books; 1988

[11] Bretherton I, Munholland K. The internal working model construct in light of contemporary neuroimaging research. In: Cassidy J, Shraver PR, editors. Handbook of Attachment: Theory, Research, and Clinical Applications. 3rd ed. New York: Guilford Press; 2016. pp. 63-88

[12] Tronick EZ. Emotions and emotional communication in infants. The American Psychologist. 1989;**44**(2):112-119. DOI: 10.1037/0003-066X.44.2.112

[13] Gianino A, Tronick EZ. The mutual regulation model: The infant's self and interactive regulation, coping, and defensive capacities. In: Field T, McCabe P, Schneiderman N, editors. Stress and Coping. Hillsdale, NJ: Erlbaum; 1988. pp. 47-68

[14] Tronick EZ. The Neurobehavioral and Social-Emotional Development of Infants and Children. New York: Norton; 2007

[15] Tronick E, Beeghly M. Infants' meaning-making and the development of mental health problems. The American Psychologist. Mar 2011;**66**(2):107-119. DOI: 10.1037/a0021631

[16] Egmose I, Cordes K, Smith-Nielsen J, Væver MS, Køppe S. Mutual regulation between infant facial affect and maternal touch in depressed and nondepressed dyads. Infant Behavior & Development. 2018;**2018**(50):274-283. DOI: 10.1016/j.infbeh.2017.05.007

[17] Banella FE, Speranza AM, Tronick E. Mutual regulation and unique forms of implicit relational knowing. Rassegna di psicologia. Nov 2018;**35**(3):67-76. DOI: 10.4458/1415-06

[18] Banella FE, Tronick E. Mutual regulation and unique forms of implicit relational knowing. In: Apter G, Devouche E, editors. Infant Psychopathology and Early Interaction: From Theories to Practice. Boston: Springer; 2019. DOI: 10.1007/978-3-030-04769-6_3

[19] Verhage ML, Schuengel C, Madigan S, Fearon RM, Oosterman M, Cassibba R, et al. Narrowing the transmission gap: A synthesis of three decades of research on intergenerational transmission of attachment. Psychological Bulletin. 2016;**142**(4):337-366. DOI: 10.1037/bul0000038

[20] Steele H, Steele M. Intergenerational patterns of attachment. In: Bartholomew K, Perlman D, editors. Attachment Processes in Adulthood. Vol. 1994. New York: The Guilford Press; 1994. pp. 93-120

[21] Crowell J, Treboux D, Gao Y, Fyffe C, Pan H, Waters E. Assessing secure base behaviour in adulthood: Development of a measure, links to adult attachment representations, and relations to couples' communication and reports of relationships. Developmental Psychology. 2002;**38**:679-693. DOI: 10.1037/0012-1649.38.5.679

[22] Fraley RC, Shaver PR. Adult romantic attachment: Theoretical developments, emerging controversies, and unanswered questions. Review of General Psychology. 2000;**4**:132-154

[23] Zajac L, Raby KL, Dozier M. Sustained effects on attachment security in middle childhood: Results from a randomized clinical trial of the Attachment and Biobehavioral Catch-up (ABC) intervention. Journal of Child Psychology and Psychiatry. 2020;**61**(4):417-424. DOI: 10.1111/jcpp.13146

[24] Bretherton I. Communication patterns, internal working models, and the intergenerational transmission of attachment relationships. Infant Mental Health Journal. 1990;**11**(3):237-252. DOI: 10.1002/1097-0355(199023)11:3<237::AID-IMHJ2280110306>3.0.CO;2-X

[25] Madigan S, Bakermans-Kranenburg MJ, Van Ijzendoorn MH, Moran G, Pederson DR, Benoit D. Unresolved states of mind, anomalous parental behavior, and disorganized attachment: A review and meta-analysis of a transmission gap. Attachment & Human Development. 2006;**8**(2):89-111. DOI: 10.1080/14616730600774458

[26] Bailey HN, Bernier A, Bouvette-Turcot A, Tarabulsy GM, Pederson DR, Becker-Stoll F. Deconstructing maternal sensitivity: Predictive relations to mother-child attachment in home and laboratory settings. Social Development. 2017;**26**:679-693

[27] Kim S, Sharp C, Carbone C. The protective role of attachment security for adolescent borderline personality disorder features via enhanced positive emotion regulation strategies. Journal of Personality Disorders. 2014;**5**(2):125-136. DOI: 10.1037/per0000038

[28] Hesse E, Main M. Second-generation effects of unresolved trauma as observed in non-maltreating parents: Dissociated, frightened, and threatening parental behavior. Psychoanalytic Inquiry. 1999;**19**:481-540

[29] Schuengel C, Bakermans-Kranenburg MJ, Van IMH. Frightening

maternal behavior linking unresolved loss and disorganized infant attachment. Journal of Consulting and Clinical Psychology. 1999;**67**:54-63

[30] Lyons-Ruth K, Yellin C, Melnick S, Atwood G. Expanding the concept of unresolved mental states: Hostile/helpless states of mind on the Adult Attachment Interview are associated with disrupted mother-infant communication and infant disorganization. Development and Psychopathology. 2005;**17**(1):1-23. DOI: 10.1017/s0954579405050017

[31] Ijzendoorn VM. Adult attachment representations, parental responsiveness, and infant attachment: A meta-analysis on the predictive validity of the Adult Attachment Interview. Psychological Bulletin. 1995;**117**(3):387-403. DOI: 10.1037/0033-2909.117.3.387

[32] Hautamäki A, Hautamäki L, Neuvonen L, Maliniemi S. Transmission of attachment across three generations: Continuity and reversal. Clinical Child Psychology and Psychiatry. 2010;**15**:347-354. DOI: 10.1177/1359104510365451

[33] Ainsworth MD, Blehar MC, Waters E, Wall S. Patterns of attachment: A psychological study of the strange situation. New York: Routledge; Lawrence Erlbaum; 1978

[34] Main M, Solomon J. Discovery of a new, insecure-disorganized/disoriented attachment pattern. In: Yogman M, Brazelton TB, editors. Affective Development in Infancy. Norwood, NJ: Ablex; 1986. pp. 95-124

[35] Main M, Solomon J. Procedures for identifying infants as disorganized/disoriented during the Ainsworth Strange Situation. In: Greenberg MT, Cicchetti D, Cummings EM, editors. Attachment in the Preschool Years. Chicago, IL: University of Chicago Press; 1990. pp. 121-160

[36] Berlin LJ, Cassidy J, Appleyard K. The influence of early attachments on other relationships. In: Cassidy J, Shaver PR, editors. Handbook of Attachment: Theory, Research, and Clinical Applications. New York: Guilford Press; 2008. pp. 333-347

[37] Mikulincer M, Shaver PR. Attachment Patterns in Adulthood: Structure, Dynamics, and Change. New York: Guilford Press; 2007

[38] Thompson RA, Goodvin R, Meyer S. Social development: Psychological understanding, self-understanding, and relationships. In: Luby JL, editor. Handbook of Preschool Mental Health: Development, Disorders, and Treatment. The Guilford Press; 2006. pp. 3-22

[39] Saunders H, Kraus A, Barone L, Biringen Z. Emotional availability: theory, research, and intervention. Frontiers in Psychology. 2015;**6**:1069. DOI: 10.3389/fpsyg.2015.01069

[40] Pascuzzo K, Cyr C, Moss E. Longitudinal association between adolescent attachment, adult romantic attachment, and emotion regulation strategies. Attachment & Human Development. 2013;**15**(1):83-103. DOI: 10.1080/14616734.2013.745713

[41] Delgado E, Sern C, Martínez I, Cruise E. Parental attachment and peer relationships in adolescence: A systematic review. International Journal of Environmental Research and Public Health. 2022;**19**(3):1064. DOI: 10.3390/ijerph19031064

[42] Saferstein JA, Neimeyer GJ, Hagans CL. Attachment as a predictor of friendship qualities in college youth. Social Behavior and Personality. 2005;**33**(8):767-776

[43] Zeifman D, Hazan C. Pair bonds as attachments: Reevaluating the evidence.

In: Cassidy J, Shaver PR, editors. Handbook of Attachment: Theory, Research, and Clinical Applications. New York: Guilford Press; 2008. p. 436

[44] Zeifman DM, Hazan C. Pair bonds as attachments: Mounting evidence in support of Bowlby's hypothesis. In: Cassidy J, Shaver PR, editors. Handbook of Attachment: Theory, Research, and Clinical Applications. 3rd ed. New York: Guilford Press; 2016

[45] Bartholomew K, Horowitz LM. Attachment styles among young adults: A test of a four-category model. Journal of Personality and Social Psychology. 1991;**61**(2):226-244. DOI: 10.1037/0022-3514.61.2.226

[46] Hazan C, Shaver P. Romantic love conceptualized as an attachment process. Journal of Personality and Social Psychology. 1987;**52**(3):511-524. DOI: 10.1037/0022-3514.52.3.511

[47] Li T, Chan D. How anxious and avoidant attachment affect romantic relationship quality differently: A meta-analytic review. European Journal of Social Psychology. 2012;**42**:406-419. DOI: 42.10.1002/ejsp.1842

[48] Simpson JA. Influence of attachment styles on romantic relationships. Journal of Personality and Social Psychology. 1990;**59**(5):971-980. DOI: 10.1037/0022-3514.59.5.971

[49] Einav M. Perceptions about parents' relationship and parenting quality, attachment styles, and young adults' intimate expectations: A cluster analytic approach. The Journal of Psychology. 2014;**148**(4):413-434. DOI: 10.1080/00223980.2013.805116

[50] Feeney J, Karantzas G. Couple conflict: Insights from an attachment perspective. Current Opinion in Psychology. 2016;**13**:60-64. DOI: 13.10.1016/j.copsyc.2016.04.017

[51] Lavy S, Mikulincer M, Shaver PR. Autonomy-proximity imbalance: An attachment theory perspective on intrusiveness in romantic relationships. Personality & Individual Differences. 2010;**48**:552-556

[52] Richter M, Schlegel K, Thomas P, Troche SJ. Adult attachment and personality as predictors of jealousy in romantic relationships. Frontiers in Psychology. 2022;**13**:861481. DOI: 10.3389/fpsyg.2022.861481

[53] Wright B, Barry M, Hughes E, Trépel D, Ali S, Allgar V, et al. Clinical effectiveness and cost-effectiveness of parenting interventions for children with severe attachment problems: A systematic review and meta-analysis. Health Technology Assessment. 2015;**19**(52):347. DOI: 10.3310/hta19520

[54] Siegal A, Levin Y, Solomon, Z. The role of attachment of each partner on marital adjustment. Journal of Family Issues. 2018;**40**(4):415-434. DOI:10.1177/0192513X18812005

[55] Barry J, Seager M, Brown B. Gender differences in the association between attachment style and adulthood relationship satisfaction (brief report). Journal of Mens Studies. 2015;**4**(3):63-74

[56] Callaci M, Vaillancourt-Morel MP, Labonté T, Brassard A, Tremblay N, Péloquin K. Attachment insecurities predicting romantic disengagement over the course of couple therapy in a naturalistic setting. Couple and Family Psychology. 2021;**10**(1):54-69. DOI: 10.1037/cfp0000158

[57] Shaver P, Hazan C. Adult romantic attachment process: Theory and evidence. In: Perlman D, Jones W, editors.

Advances in Personal Relationships Outcomes. London: Jessica Kingsley Publisher; 1992. pp. 29-70

[58] Thompson RA, Simpson JA, Berlin LJ. Taking perspective on attachment theory and research: Nine fundamental questions. Attachment & Human Development. 2022;**24**(5):543-560. DOI: 10.1080/14616734.2022.2030132

[59] Feeney JA, Noller P, Callan VJ. Attachment style, communication and satisfaction in the early years of marriage. In: Bartholomew K, Perlman D, editors. Attachment Processes in Adulthood. London: Jessica Kingsley Publishers; 1994. pp. 269-308

[60] Waters TE, Magro SW, Alhajeri J, Yang R, Groh A, et al. Early child care experiences and attachment representations at age 18 years: Evidence from the NICHD study of Early Child Care and Youth Development. Developmental Psychology. 2021;**57**(4):548-556. DOI: 10.1037/dev0001165

[61] Kobak RR, Hazan C. Attachment in marriage: Effects of security and accuracy of working models. Journal of Personality and Social Psychology. *1991*;*60*(6):861-869. DOI: 10.1037/0022-3514.60.6.861

[62] Bartholomew K. Avoidance of intimacy: An attachment perspective. Journal of Social and Personal Relationships. 1990;**7**(2):147-178. DOI: 10.1177/0265407590072001

[63] Pietromonaco PR, Carnelley KB. Gender and working models of attachment: Consequences for perceptions of self and romantic relationships. Personal Relationships. 1994;**1**(1):63-82. DOI: 10.1111/j.1475-6811.1994.tb00055.x

[64] Levine A, Heller R. Attached: The New Science of Adult Attachment and How It Can Help You Find- and Keep-Love. New York: Jeremy P. Tarcher/Penguin; 2011

[65] Senchak M, Leonard KE. Attachment styles and marital adjustment among newlywed couples. Journal of Social and Personal Relationships. 1992;**9**(1):51-64. DOI: 10.1177/0265407592091003

[66] Holmes BM, Johnson KR. Adult attachment and romantic partner preference: A review. Journal of Social and Personal Relationships. 2009;**26**:833-852. DOI: 10.1177/0265407509345653

[67] O'Leary KD. Physical aggression between spouses: A social learning theory perspective. In: Van Hasselt VB, Morrison RL, Bellack AS, Hersen M, editors. Handbook of Family Violence. New York: Plenum Press; 1988. pp. 31-55

[68] Whitton SW, Rhoades GK, Stanley SM, Markman HJ. Effects of parental divorce on marital commitment and confidence. Journal of Family Psychology. 2008;**22**:789-793. DOI: 10.1037/a0012800

[69] Wampler K, Shi L, Nelson B, Kimball T. The adult attachment interview and observed couple interaction: Implications for an intergenerational perspective on couple therapy. Family Process. 2003;**42**:497-515

[70] Knapp DJ, Norton AM, Sandberg JG. Family-of-origin, relationship self-regulation, and attachment in marital relationships. Contemporary Family Therapy. 2015;**37**:130-141

[71] Gardner B, Busby D, Burr B, Lyon S. Getting to the root of relationship attributions: Family-of-origin perspectives on self and partner

views. Contemporary Family Therapy. 2011;**33**:253-272. DOI: 10.1007/s10591-011-9163-5

[72] Gleeson G, Fitzgerald A. Exploring the association between adult attachment styles in romantic relationships, perceptions of parents from childhood and relationship satisfaction. Health. 2014;**6**:1643-1661. DOI: 10.4236/health.2014.613196

[73] Mikulincer M, Shaver PR. Attachment in Adulthood. 2nd ed. New York: Guilford Press; 2016

[74] Mondor J, McDuff P, Lussier Y, Wright J. Couples in therapy: Actor-partner analyses of the relationships between adult romantic attachment and marital satisfaction. American Journal of Family Therapy. 2011;**39**:112-123. DOI: 10.1080/01926187.2010.530163

[75] Boisvert MM, Wright J, Tremblay N, McDuff P. Couples' reports of relationship problems in a naturalistic therapy setting. The Family Journal. 2011;**19**(4):362-368

[76] Halford WK, Pepping CA. What every therapist needs to know about couple therapy. Behaviour Change. 2019;**36**(3):121-142

[77] Feeney JA. Hurt feelings in couple relationships: Exploring the role of attachment and perceptions of personal injury. Personal Relationships. 2005;**12**(2):253-271. DOI: 10.1111/j.1350-4126.2005.00114.x

[78] Johnson SM. Couple and family therapy: An attachment perspective. In: Cassidy J, Shaver PR, editors. Handbook of Attachment: Theory, Research, and Clinical Applications. New York, NY: Guilford Press; 2008. pp. 811-829

[79] Simpson JA, Rholes WS. Adult attachment, stress, and romantic relationships. Current Opinion in Psychology. 2017;**13**:19-24. DOI: 10.1016/j.copsyc.2016.04.006

[80] Burke E, Danquah A, Berry K. A qualitative exploration of the use of attachment theory in adult psychological therapy. Clinical Psychology & Psychotherapy. 2015;**23**(2):142-154. DOI: 23.10.1002/cpp.1943

[81] Bifulco A, Moran PM, Ball C, Bernazzani O. Adult attachment style. I: Its relationship to clinical depression. Social Psychiatry and Psychiatric Epidemiology. 2002;**37**(2):50-59. DOI: 10.1007/s127-002-8215-0

[82] Berry K, Barrowclough C, Wearden A. Attachment theory: A framework for understanding symptoms and interpersonal relationships in psychosis. Behaviour Research and Therapy. 2008;**46**(12):1275-1282. DOI: 10.1016/j.brat.2008.08.009

[83] Petersen J, Le B. Psychological distress, attachment, and conflict resolution in romantic relationships. Modern Psychological Studies. 2017:**23**. Available from: https://scholar.utc.edu/mps/vol23/iss1/3

[84] Hicks AM, Diamond LM. Don't go to bed angry: Attachment, conflict, and affective and physiological reactivity. Personal Relationships. 2011;**18**(2):266-284. DOI: 10.1111/j.1475-6811.2011.01355.x

[85] Carnelley KB, Pietromonaco PR, Jaffe K. Depression, working models of others, and relationship functioning. Journal of Personality and Social Psychology. 1994;**66**:127-140

[86] Collins NL, Read SJ. Adult attachment, working models, and

relationship quality in dating couples. Journal of Personality and Social Psychology. 1990;**58**(4):644-663. DOI: 10.1037/0022-3514.58.4.644

[87] Cozzarelli C, Karafa JA, Collins NL, Tagler MJ. Stability and change in adult attachment styles: Associations with personal vulnerabilities, life events, and global construals of self and others. Journal of Social and Clinical Psychology. 2003;**22**(3):315-346. DOI: 10.1521/jscp.22.3.315.22888

[88] Pinquart M, Feußner C, Ahnert L. Meta-analytic evidence for stability in attachments from infancy to early adulthood. Attachment & Human Development. 2013;**15**(2):189-218. DOI: 10.1080/14616734.2013.746257

[89] Zhang F, Labouvie-Vief G. Stability and fluctuation in attachment style over a 6-year period. Attachment & Human Development. 2005;**6**(4):419-437. DOI: 10.1080/1461673042000303127

[90] Waters E, Merrick S, Treboux D, Crowell J, Albersheim L. Attachment security in infancy and early adulthood: A twenty-year longitudinal study. Child Development. 2000;**71**(3):684-689. DOI: 10.1111/1467-8624.00176

[91] Gillath O, Hart JJ. The effects of psychological security and insecurity on political attitudes and leadership preferences. European Journal of Social Psychology. 2010;**40**:122-134

[92] McClure MJ, Bartz JA, Lydon JE. Uncovering and overcoming ambivalence: The role of chronic and contextually activated attachment in two-person social dilemmas. Journal of Personality. 2013;**81**(1):103-117. DOI: 10.1111/j.1467-6494.2012.00788.x

[93] Mikulincer M, Hirschberger G, Nachmias O, Gillath O. The affective component of the secure base schema: Affective priming with representations of attachment security. Journal of Personality and Social Psychology. 2001;**81**(2):305-321. DOI: 10.1037/0022-3514.81.2.305

[94] Mikulincer M, Shaver PR, Sahdra BK, Bar-On N. Can security-enhancing interventions overcome psychological barriers to responsiveness in couple relationships? Attachment & Human Development. 2013;**15**(3):246-260. DOI: 10.1080/14616734.2013.782653

[95] Mikulincer M, Gillath O, Halevy V, Avihou N, Avidan S, Eshkoli N. Attachment theory and reactions to others' needs: Evidence that activation of the sense of attachment security promotes empathic responses. Journal of Personality and Social Psychology. 2001;**81**:1205-1224

[96] Carnelley K, Rowe A. Repeated priming of attachment security influences later views of self and relationships. Personal Relationships. 2007;**14**:307-320. DOI: 10.1111/j.1475-6811.2007.00156.x

[97] Hudson NW, Fraley RC. Does attachment anxiety promote the encoding of false memories? An investigation of the processes linking adult attachment to memory errors. Journal of Personality and Social Psychology. 2018;**115**(4):688-715. DOI: 10.1037/pspp0000215

[98] Johnson SM, Whiffen VE. Made to measure: Adapting emotionally focused couple therapy to partners' attachment styles. Clinical Psychologist. 1999;**6**(4):366-381. DOI: 10.1093/clipsy.6.4.366/

[99] Rehman U, Holtzworth-Munroe A. A cross-cultural examination of the relation of marital communication

behaviour to marital satisfaction. Journal of Family Psychology. 2008;**21**:759-763. DOI: 10.1037/0893-3200.21.4.759

[100] Wills RM. Insight Oriented Marital Therapy [Treatment Manual]. Detroit: Wayne State University; 1982

[101] Jacobson NS, Margolin G. Marital Therapy: Strategies Based on Social Learning And Behaviour Exchange Principles. New York: Brunner/Mazel; 1979

[102] Christensen LL, Russell CS, Miller RB, Peterson CM. The process of change in couples therapy: A qualitative investigation. Journal of Marital and Family Therapy. 1998;**24**(2):177-188. DOI: 10.1111/j.1752-0606.1998.tb01074.x

[103] Snyder DK, Halford WK. Evidence-based couple therapy: Current status and future directions. Journal of Family Therapy. 2012;**34**(3):229-249. DOI: 10.1111/j.1467-6427.2012.00599.x

[104] Wiebe S, Johnson SM. A review of the research in emotionally focused therapy for couples. Family Process. 2016;**55**(3):390-407. DOI: 10.1111/famp.12229

[105] Havaasi N, Zahra KK, Mohsen ZF. Compare the efficacy of emotion focused couple therapy and Gottman couple therapy method in marital burnout and changing conflict resolution styles. Journal of Fundamentals of Mental Health. 2018;**20**(1):15-25

[106] Byrne M, Carr A, Clarke. The efficacy of behavioural couples therapy and emotionally focused therapy for couple distress. Contemporary Family Therapy. 2004;**26**(4):361-387

[107] Ahmadi FS, Zarei E, Fallahchai SR. The effectiveness of emotionally-focused couple therapy in resolution of marital conflicts between the couples who visited the consultation centers. Journal of Educational and Management Studies. 2014;**4**(1):118-123

[108] Johnson LN, Tambling RB, Mennenga KD, Ketring SA, Oka M, Anderson SR, et al. Examining attachment avoidance and attachment anxiety across eight sessions of couple therapy. Journal of Marital and Family Therapy. 2016;**42**(2):195-212

[109] Wiebe SA, Johnson SM, Lafontaine MF, Moser MB, Dalgleish TL, Tasca GA. Two-year follow-up outcomes in emotionally focused couple therapy: An investigation of relationship satisfaction and attachment trajectories. Journal of Marital and Family Therapy. 2017;**43**(2):227-244

[110] Moser MB, Johnson SM, Dalgleish TL, Wiebe SA, Tasca GA. The impact of blamer-softening on romantic attachment in emotionally focused couples therapy. Journal of Marital and Family Therapy. 2018;**44**(4):640-654

[111] Moser MB, Johnson SM, Dalgleish TL, Lafontaine MF, Wiebe SA, Tasca GA. Changes in relationship-specific attachment in emotionally focused couple therapy. Journal of Marital and Family Therapy. 2016;**42**(2):231-245. DOI: 10.1111/jmft.12139

[112] Rostami M, Taheri A, Abdi M, Kermani N. The effectiveness of instructing emotion-focused approach in improving the marital satisfaction in couples. Procedia - Social and Behavioral Sciences. 2014;**114**:693-698. DOI: 10.1016/j.sbspro.2013.12.769

[113] Benson LA, Sevier M, Christensen A. The impact of behavioral couple therapy on attachment in distressed couples. Journal of Marital and Family Therapy. 2013;**39**(4):407-420. DOI: 10.1111/jmft.12020

[114] Naama SC. Evaluation of the clinical efficacy of Emotionally Focused Couples Therapy on psychological adjustment and natural killer cell cytotoxicity in early breast cancer. Doctoral Dissertation. 2008. Retrieved from Library and Archives Canada.

[115] Weissman N, Batten SV, Rheem KD, Wiebe SA, Potts RM, Barone M, et al. The effectiveness of emotionally focused couples therapy with veterans with PTSD: A pilot study. Journal of Couple and Relationship Therapy. 2017;**17**(1): 25-41. DOI: 10.1080/15332691.2017.1285261/

[116] Wittenborn AK, Liu T, Ridenour TA, Lachmar EM, Mitchell EA, Seedall RB. Randomized controlled trial of emotionally focused couple therapy compared to treatment as usual for depression: Outcomes and mechanisms of change. Journal of Marital and Family Therapy. 2018;**2018**:45. DOI: 10.1111/jmft.12350

[117] Stith SM, Rosen KH, McCollum EE. Effectiveness of couples treatment for spouse abuse. Journal of Marital and Family Therapy. 2003;**29**(3):407-426. DOI: 10.1111/j.1752-0606.2003.tb01215.x

[118] Solelmanl AA, Najafi M, Ahmadi K, Javidl N, Hoselnl Kamkar E, Mahboubl M. The effectiveness of emotionally focused couples therapy on sexual satisfaction and marital adjustment of infertile couples with marital conflicts. International Journal of Fertility and Sterility. 2015;**9**(3):393-402

[119] Huang CY, Sirikantraporn S, Pichayayothin NB, Turner-Cobb JM. Parental attachment, adult-child romantic attachment, and marital satisfaction: An examination of cultural context in Taiwanese and Thai heterosexual couples. International Journal of Environmental Research and Public Health. 21 Jan 2020;**17**(3):692. DOI: 10.3390/ijerph17030692

[120] Liu TI, Wittenborn AN. Emotionally focused therapy with culturally diverse couples. In: Furrow JL, Johnson SM, Bradley BA, editors. The Emotionally Focused Casebook: New Directions in Treating Couples. New York: Routledge; 2011. pp. 295-316

[121] Poursardar F, Sadeghi M, Goodarzi C, Roozbehani M. Comparing the efficacy of emotionally Focused Couple Therapy and integrative Behavioral Couple Therapy in improving the symptoms of emotional regulation in couples with marital conflict. Journal of Mazandaran University of Medical Sciences. 2019;**29**(173):50-63

[122] Benson LA, McGinn MM, Christensen A. Common principles of couple therapy. Behavior Therapy. 2012;***43***(1):25-35. DOI: 10.1016/j.beth.2010.12.009

[123] Gottman JM, Gottman JS. Gottman method couple therapy. In: Gurman AS, editor. Clinical Handbook of Couple Therapy. New York: The Guilford Press; 2008. pp. 138-164